THE NURSING PROCESS

assessing, planning,
implementing, evaluating

Second Edition

HELEN YURA, PH.D., R.N.

Consultant in Nursing Education
Department of Baccalaureate and Higher Degree Programs
National League for Nursing.
Formerly Chairman, Department of Nursing
St. Joseph College
Emmitsburg, Maryland

MARY B. WALSH, M.S.N., R.N.

Assistant Professor
Medical and Surgical Nursing
The Catholic University of America
Washington, D.C.

THE
NURSING
PROCESS

assessing, planning, implementing, evaluating

Second Edition

APPLETON-CENTURY-CROFTS / New York
A Publishing Division of Prentice-Hall, Inc.

Library of Congress Cataloging in Publication Data

Yura, Helen
  The nursing process, second edition

  First ed. (1967) edited by H. Yura and M.B. Walsh and
entered under Catholic University of America School of
Nursing.
  Bibliography: pp. 197-209
  1. Nurses and nursing—Congresses. I. Walsh, Mary B., joint
author. II. Catholic University of America. School of Nursing. The nursing process. III. Title. [DNLM: 1. Nurse-patient
relations—Congresses. 2. Nursing—Congresses. WY100 N976
1973]
RT3.Y87 1973   610.73   73-11004
ISBN 0-8385-7031-3

74 75 76 77 78 79 / 10 9 8 7 6 5 4 3

Library of Congress Catalog Card Number 73–11004

PRINTED IN THE UNITED STATES OF AMERICA 0–8385–7031–3

*This book
is dedicated to
our families*

Preface

The purpose of this book is to update data on the nursing process, data which we edited in 1967. The information presented in the seven papers of the 1967 Continuing Education Series at the Catholic University are incorporated in this book, which also includes pertinent data developed since the 1967 publication. A selective, though not exhaustive, review of the literature related to as well as concepts and ideas about the nursing process which are of value to the baccalaureate nursing student are presented. Our views on the process are explained, and our philosophies and convictions about nursing are emphasized. The nursing setting is not limited to any one environment—home, clinic, hospital, or other agency—instead, we suggest uses of the nursing process in any setting in which there is a client, actual or potential. Several illustrations of the application of the nursing process will be presented; these can act as guides to those who use this book for teaching and learning purposes. We hope to stimulate ideas, activate thoughts and initiate actions.

This book is divided into five chapters: Chapter 1 briefly reviews the historic background and current ideas of the nursing process. Chapter 2 reviews some of the theories fundamental to and related to the nursing process. Chapter 3 analyzes and discusses phases of the process; chapter 4 suggests applications; and chapter 5 identifies future potentials in terms of study and research. A suggested reading list appears at the end of the book.

The word *client*, as used throughout this text, refers to an individual or family. It is our belief that nursing is practised in many settings, with a variety of consumers, few of whom possess a simple problem and all with some family, or at least significant person, concerned about them. Some consumers may have potential problems; the nurse must help the individual stay well. Some clients will have actual problems; the nurse's role is to help them to return to a state as normal for them as possible. The authors believe that the word *client* conveys this multifaceted concept of the consumer of nursing.

To facilitate readability, the pronoun *she* refers to the nurse; *he* refers to the client. No bias is intended in this use of pronouns; we trust our readers will understand and agree with us.

As the number of nurses who publish ideas and concepts about their profession increases, so does agreement about what nursing is and what the goals of nursing action are. Numerous nurses share the person-centered, goal-directed focus of their practice. In many instances, it is impossible to cite original ideas, for ours are molded and developed by the thoughts and ideas of many. Only a few specific ideas or particular contributions are cited in the text; this does not reflect the total number of nurses who have contributed. Many nurses will read their own ideas and convictions into those presented, since they undoubtedly developed these at the same time as the authors. We find it a positive indication that, in our discussions and in the literature, there is increasing evidence that nurses agree about our *raison d'etre*. This trend toward unified thinking among professional nurses reinforces the value of the nursing process as the core of nursing practice.

Were it not for the challenge and stimulation given by students with whom we have been associated for many years, this book would not have been possible. Our fellow faculty and our colleagues in nursing service stimulated ideas and encouraged us with their positive response to our development of the nursing process. We extend our appreciation to each of these persons and say: "Without you, this could not have been done!"

We are especially grateful to Ruth Lowe for her secretarial assistance, to Gloria Selitto who typed the manuscript, and to Ralph Selitto who drew the illustrations.

Helen Yura
Mary Walsh

Contents

THE NURSING PROCESS

assessing, planning,
implementing, evaluating

Second Edition

chapter one

Development of the Nursing Process

The nursing process is central to all nursing actions; it is the very essence of nursing, applicable in any setting, in any frame of reference, and within any philosophy. It is flexible and adaptable, adjustable to a number of variables, yet sufficiently structured so as to provide a base from which many nursing actions can proceed. Phases and subphases within the process can be examined, analyzed, and pursued deliberately by the nurse as she provides for clients with whom she functions.

HISTORIC EVENTS IN NURSING AND THE NURSING PROCESS

To better portray the nursing process, some reflection on certain historic events will be of benefit. The exact time period of each era is neither distinct nor precise, but the progress and developments which have had a major impact in nursing can be grouped as follows:

1. Events preceding World War II
2. Events during World War II

3. Events following World War II
   a. During the First 20 post-war years
   b. During the past decade

Events Preceding World War II

In the days of the early Christians, the practice of nursing was based on unselfishness and love of neighbor; there was concern for meeting the needs of each sick person. The actions of persons who practiced nursing were directed toward helping the sick get well so that he or she could lead a healthier and happier life. Persons who practiced nursing received little formal education. Most nursing behavior was learned by the apprenticeship system; the person who wanted to be a nurse accompanied an experienced practitioner—a role model—whose behavior was copied or imitated. Much nursing action depended on the judgments of experienced practitioners.

A history of people who lived in the middle ages reports that many persons cared for the sick; these were persons who responded to the social forces prevalent at the time—through their concern for people—to meet the basic human needs of the sick. During the last two centuries of this medieval period, there were many changes in national, political, and social structures, all associated with the unrest and turmoil that necessarily accompany major change.[1]

As social forces and political structures changed, so did the practice of nursing; history records many phases through which nursing proceeded and survived, with many ups and downs along the way. It was not until the days of Florence Nightingale (1820-1910) that nursing began to take on some semblance of structure, some effort toward deliberate actions. In today's language, Florence Nightingale would have been called a *militant*; there was little *establishment* with which to disagree, yet she questioned traditions and customs that had been accepted for many years. She set about designing her own rules, and ran a very "tight ship" to achieve what she judged necessary to provide the best care for patients. Despite her maverick nature, she was far-sighted and set admirable goals, establishing some firm foundations on which nursing continues to rest today. She emphasized knowledge, suggesting that the preparation needed by the staff nurse is different from that needed by a supervisor or administrator. She also was concerned about just remuneration for nurses, although the 12-hour work day, the 7-day work week, and the 5-cent raise after a 6-month probationary period cannot compare with the work demands and pay of the mid-twentieth century. Regretfully, Florence Nightingale did not think kindly of male nurses, nor did she emphasize or talk about the nursing process; nevertheless, she deserves her title as the founder of modern nursing; she placed nursing on a respected and respectable level.[2]

During the years between Florence Nightingale's efforts and the beginning of World War II, there was little progress in nursing. These years can be called *the era of maintenance*, or *the era of little or no change*. This was a time of complacency in nursing; World War I and the economic depression were among the reasons. Other professions, as well as nursing, experienced similar lags in progress and merely maintained their status quo.

Events During World War II

The conflict of World War II was a propelling force behind many changes in the world. During this post-depression era the need for technology increased. The health professions, especially nursing, also felt the impact of this technologic change. War casualties increased the need for physicians and nurses; pressures of war and feelings of patriotism created different ways to cope with human needs; the relatively uncomplicated triad of *Doctor-Nurse-Client* gave way to a multidimensional health team, the dimensions of which have continued to grow and expand.

The contributions of medical corpsmen during the war set the pattern for auxiliary personnel in the health professions. Because knowledge grew and accumulated rapidly, it was soon obvious that more persons would be needed to cope with the challenges. Advances in clinical medicine, such as early ambulation; changes and advances in the treatment of burns; and the discovery of new drugs, especially antibiotics, were all forerunners to the changes that occurred in nursing.

Events Following World War II
During the First 20 Post-War Years

The two decades that followed V-J Day brought more areas of change more rapidly than did any other period in the history of nursing. Health care systems in the United States were viewed differently after the war. The public became more aware of what constitutes good health care; the population increased markedly, the economy changed and grew, and there was a trend toward urbanization, an explosion of scientific knowledge, an acceleration of medical discoveries, new methods of therapy, new inventions, and finally the recognition that it is just as important to keep people well as it is to treat illness. After World War II an effort was made to move more deliberately and more creatively; the impact of this movement continues to be felt with increasing intensity.

As knowledge increased and the economy changed, there were new developments on the educational scene. The GI Bill of Rights provided money so that many veterans could prepare for a career or job for which they had never hoped to qualify. Nursing as well as other schools were flooded with applicants for degrees. Education was changing the art and practice of nursing. A theme heard frequently during the postwar era was: *the nurse must give total patient care.* Nurses were to be all things to their clients. Even though other health team members appeared on the scene, nurses were reluctant to give up the idea of *total patient care*, or perhaps they did not know how to give up those aspects of care which were not nursing. The scene began to change and the nurse learned that team work was the name of the new game. It was not easy for her to relinquish the idea that she had to be all things to all clients. Gradually emphasis shifted, and although the nurse continued to be aware of the totality of the individual her role was altered to include working cooperatively with other members of the health team who also were concerned with the client's care and welfare. The functions of referring clients to other disciplines and communicating with each was the nurse's responsibility; she continued her concept of total patient care, but implementing the concept was considered to be the responsibility of all members of the health team, including the nurse.

The war precipitated changes during the early forties, and the later years of this decade witnessed a concerned nursing profession. The health care system was struggling with the increased numbers of personnel that had been introduced into it; efforts were made to define the roles of each to prevent duplication, yet retain what each person, or each group, felt was the essence of nursing. The turmoil created by the changes everyone was experiencing was culminated, in the profession of nursing, by asking a nonnurse to provide an unbiased assessment of the status of the profession and to suggest ways in which it could move constructively. The report presented by Esther Lucile Brown in 1948 was a major turning point in the lives of nurses and nursing.[3] The groundwork provided by the recommendations of this report has been the basis for many of the changes that have occurred in nursing during this past quarter century, and for some recommendations that the profession continues to strive for.

As did Florence Nightingale, Esther Brown expressed her concern for adequate remuneration of nurses for quality service. Noteworthy is the fact that the discussion of remuneration seldom stands alone; it is usually coupled with the responsibility for providing quality service. This concern is as true today as it was in the days of Florence Nightingale, and is one of the major justifications for employing the nursing process. Through organized and deliberate nursing action, quality care is more certain, and the means for evaluating the quality of care are provided.

During the 1950s, after the Brown report was published, attention was focused on the appropriate use of the term *professional*, rapidly expanding health programs, and the working relationship between the nurse and allied health personnel for the benefit of the client.

For many years professionalism had been discussed and

whether nursing met the criteria for a profession had been debated. Several authors suggested criteria for a profession; those set forth by Flexner[4] were quoted frequently. More recently, several sociologists have identified the variables operating in the attempts to define professionalism and to establish criteria basic to professions. Schein has presented a composite of these efforts and has defined ten criteria of professions, all of which are appropriate to the profession of nursing.[5] Nurses continue to be concerned that nursing meet these criteria; however, current emphasis is focused on nursing action and on the client—the recipient of nursing, rather than on the nurse who does or is the agent of nursing. Whether or not others agree, nurses now accept the idea that nursing is a profession; they do not debate it. And as a group of professionals, the nurse's major concern is to provide quality care for clients; her energies are devoted to determining how to provide this care.

In a continuing effort to establish nursing as a profession, various approaches were used. During the latter part of the fifties, attempts were made to define nursing functions. When nursing actions were discussed, a number of crucial questions were posed, such as: To what extent do a nurse's actions affect people? How significant are the nurse's decisions and judgments to the present and future welfare of the service consumer? How complex are these actions in terms of the nurse's education and experience? Is there ample and appropriate knowledge available to and used by the nurse as a basis for her acts? Is there some check on the effectiveness of her actions? Does her performance improve with experience and does she modify her plans according to available knowledge and experience? Is the consumer able to judge the effectiveness of a nursing action? He can judge it in terms of his own needs, but is this the only measure available to him? How does a specific act measure up to those actions of other nurses?[6]

Inherent within these questions and criteria is the pertinent observation that a code of ethics is both important and essential. The fact that this code[7] exists is important since it meets one criterion for a profession and is reflected in the nurse's actions. More important than the mere existence of the code is its use as a basis for sound action by the nurse.

Events Following World War II
During the Past Decade

Although the literature teems with materials about nursing, the question is still asked: What is nursing? Perhaps the answer is so obvious, a precise definition is unnecessary or the many variables operant make a precise definition impossible. Most nursing texts published recently contain at least one sizeable section in which nursing is defined as it is conceived by the author(s). Nurses appear ready to accept, respect, and expect nurse-authors as well as nurse-practitioners to present their individual definitions and concepts about nursing.

When the structure of society was less complex than it is today, the intuitive functioning of the nurse was usually adequate to provide care. A well-intentioned, well-meaning person with an innate ability to care for the sick was an excellent person to help the person who was ill. Even in that uncomplicated day, however, each person had a different mental image of the term *nursing*. Today, a number of variables determine the complexion of this image, ranging from the actions of a mother surrogate to a top-level administrator. The discussion of *what is nursing* can be approached from any one of a number of avenues. Nursing can be defined or discussed according to: the actions used in performing the service; the roles of the persons who do the nursing; the functions of the nurse; the consumer's image of nursing; the image of nursing that nursing peers have; the philosophy of nursing as perceived by practitioners; the settings where nursing is performed; the value placed on the individual who needs nursing; respect for the client viewed from the employer-employee standpoint. These are examples of avenues or points from which one can begin to discuss or to define nursing. These potential areas are mentioned to emphasize the complex nature of nursing.

The nurse today faces the challenge of many kinds of

nurses as well as increasing numbers of health-related or paramedical personnel. Specialties within the health team have risen to meteoric proportions and are still rising. Increasing the complexity of nursing are the different types of educational programs in which nurses are prepared. The diploma program has yielded to baccalaureate programs, associate degree programs, and some variations of each in terms of the length of each program and its expected goal. Any group of nurses, functioning in a setting where nursing is practiced, will probably contain representatives from each of these programs. Coping with each other in carrying out the nursing process is another of the challenges confronting nursing and nurses; it is not an easy task to cope with many differently prepared nurses.

Knowledge continues to grow at a faster pace than it did during the immediate post-war years. Technology and computers, changes in education, and the space age have had an overwhelming impact on the forward momentum of advances and changes in today's society. The layman began to be heard more clearly after the world survived the war of the forties. The public is becoming knowledgeable, learning more and more about his health, his illnesses, and his rights; and this vocal client is not only presenting new challenges to the health professions, but is creating a need for new approaches to health care, emphasizing the need for preventive medicine as well as therapeutic care during sickness.

One of the major events of the sixties was the publication of the *American Nurses' Association's First Position on Education for Nursing.* Although not yet fully implemented, the position paper has initiated much discussion and many debates, as well as a definite trend in nursing. Essentially, the position of the American Nurses' Association is that the education of persons who practice nursing should take place in institutions of higher education; the professional nurse should be prepared in baccalaureate programs of nursing; the technical nurse in associate degree programs; and the assistant in the health services should be prepared in preservice programs in vocational education institutions rather than in on-the-job training programs.[8] The appearance and implementation of this position paper provided the impetus for accepting the nursing process as a deliberate, systematic, and organized manner of performing nursing practice.

Another significant event was the appointment, in 1961, by the Surgeon General of the U.S. Public Health Service, of a Consultant Group on Nursing who were to provide advice about nursing needs and problems in the United States. The group operated on the basis that nursing is an essential element in health care, and that public understanding and support will be necessary to solve problems in nursing. Though concerned about an increasing demand for nurses, the need for quality in nursing education, nursing service, and nursing research was constantly emphasized. The group identified needs and set goals for nursing during the 1970s.[9] The recommendations of this study led to the appointment of a National Commission for the Study of Nursing and Nursing Education. The appointed Commissioners met for the first time in 1967. A comprehensive and in-depth study resulted from the efforts of the people on this commission; they pursued three areas—nursing roles and functions, nursing education, and professional growth and development. Specific recommendations are contained in the report related to increased research, altered educational patterns, and enhanced support for nursing.[10] The efforts of the Consultant Group and the Commissioners further emphasize the importance of pursuing nursing in a systematic way, hence the significance of the deliberate use of the nursing process.

History records significant events in the development of nursing, and these can be grouped into the events that occurred before, during, and after World War II. Nursing moved from a humanitarian caring for the sick, through a period of complacency, and survived the acceleration of all facets of life and living as well as changes in the health scene that were precipitated by and followed World War II. The Brown Report in 1948, the ANA Position Paper in 1965, the report of the Surgeon General's Consultant Group, and the report of the National Commission in 1970 are major events that have stimulated changes in nursing. Having lived through efforts to prove that nursing is a profession, and having survived verbal barrages in attempts to define nursing and what is unique about it, the profession is now in the throes of defining the concepts, theories, and science of nursing. This is the dictum of the 1970s.

DEFINITIONS OF NURSING

More recent trends have moved from the debate about whether or not nursing is a profession to concern for a systematic determination of the essence of nursing. Definitions, concepts, and theories of nursing are appearing with increasing frequency. These efforts suggest a qualitative, deliberate approach to thorough analysis and study of the whole of nursing. Such constructive efforts, pursued by a variety of nurses over a period of time, will provide the nursing profession with the structural framework within which the process and knowledge of nursing can be examined, analyzed critically, revised, and improved continually in a sound scientific manner.

A number of nurses have defined nursing; some have defined a concept of nursing, others have stated beliefs about nursing, and still others have defined a philosophy of nursing. Important data about these subjects can be found in publications about the role and function of nurses; these are all attempts to state the essence of nursing.

Some nurses have contributed to the efforts made to define nursing, each developing and making a statement as to what nursing is according to her own philosophy, education, and experience. Throughout these efforts to define the unique function of nursing, various authors have expressed, in different words, what they see as the function and role of nursing. It is apparent that there is something different about nursing than the service provided by other disciplines. Although many nurses have developed definitions of nursing independently of each other, the various presentations convey similar ideas but use different words and various frames of reference. Individual philosophies are apparent in each definition and values come through; one can determine the extent to which a client is viewed as a person and the extent to which he is respected as an individual with human needs and human rights. These are all guides used by the nurse to define and report what it is she finds important in nursing.

Several selected definitions and discussions of nursing are presented here to illustrate the development of ideas about nursing.

One of the earliest definitions of nursing was presented in 1943 by Sister Olivia Gowan, a far-sighted pioneer in nursing education. Sister viewed nursing, in its broadest sense, as an art and science involving the total patient; promoting spiritual, mental, and physical health; stressing health education and health preservation; ministering to the sick; caring for the patient's environment; giving health service to the family, the community, and the individual.[11] This definition appeared in print long before it was "fashionable" to define nursing, and the comprehensive definition of nursing by Sister Olivia was, for many years, the one most accepted and most often quoted.

An article in *Nursing Outlook* in 1957 in which Frances Reiter Kreuter[12] discussed good nursing care is frequently referred to by nurses. Kreuter's contributions have continued to appear in print to the present time. Certain themes and concepts are evident as one reads her material. Paramount is her vision of the nurse as the mother surrogate. Not all nurses agree with this terminology, but if one analyzes Erikson's identification of the developmental phases of childhood and the role of the parent in each phase, the term *mother surrogate* becomes more acceptable. For example: a basic tenet in teaching a child is to gain his or her trust; so too, trust in the nurse is the basis for the client care she provides. A child learns independence gradually; the mother teaches him and helps him to become independent as he grows and develops. Developing initiative is fostered and encouraged by the mother so the child can progress to the limit of his capacity or ability.[13] These findings can be applied to the role of nurse and client in which Kreuter sees the nurse as protecting the patient, teaching him, performing for him those acts of self-care he cannot do himself, and providing comfort and encouragement. Although she calls these "ministrations," they can be viewed also as nursing actions—ministering to basic needs, administering, observing, teaching, supervising, or guiding, planning with, and communicating with the patient. Kreuter also discusses direct care, in which the nurse gives direct physical care, and indirect care, in which she engages in activities that do not bring her into immediate contact with the client. Some nurses agree with these concepts in their entirety; some agree with them partially; nevertheless, Kreuter has made major contributions to the development of concepts of nursing through numerous and thought-provoking materials.

Dorothy Johnson's presentations have also precipitated thought and discussion among nurses. Central to her thesis is the idea that all health workers have something unique to offer the client, but how to determine that which is uniquely nursing is what concerns nurses. To cope with the client's problems, each person sees certain nursing problems that require assessment, decision, and action.[14]

To intellectualize the discussion about nursing, Dr. Johnson suggested, more than a decade ago, that nursing is a direct service to persons under stress relative to their basic human needs.[14] Nursing effort and actions are focused on relieving tension and discomfort so as to restore or maintain the internal and interpersonal equilibrium. This equilibrium is a dynamic and transitional state in which stability is a delicately balanced component. Once stability is achieved, constant adjustment and effort are necessary to maintain it. The activities in which nurses are engaged for the benefit of the client should contribute to the goal of equilibrium.[15]

In 1963, Ernestine Wiedenbach contributed additional ideas to the nursing literature. She identified the purpose of nursing as meeting the requirements of persons experiencing some need for help. Three major units of nursing practice were identified: (a) recognizing a person's need for help, (b) giving or ministering that help, and (c) validating that the help given was the help needed. The heart of nursing was seen as helping others; due concern was expressed for the nurse's feelings and thoughts as well as for those of the client experiencing the problem. Essentially, emphasis was placed on the interpersonal aspect of actions that are nursing, and on identifying the behavioral stimulus for the person in need so as to designate the actions to take. The purpose of nursing was identified as "facilitating the efforts of the individual to overcome obstacles which interfere with his ability to respond capably to demands made of him by his condition, environment, situation, and time."[16]

Although she identified her ideas and concepts much earlier than 1966, in this year Virginia Henderson's book, *The Nature of Nursing*, contributed data to the increasing growth of information about nursing. Certain ideas and thoughts were distinctive about Miss Henderson's writings. She urged each nurse to define, for herself, what she sees nursing to be and to develop her own concept, rather than merely imitate others or act under authority. The nurse was viewed as an independent practitioner, helping the client to perform those activities he cannot perform unaided at the moment. Miss Henderson was one of the few persons to include in her definition the idea that efforts to return the client to a state of wellness are not always successful. She recognized that unless a nurse is realistic about the probable or possible negative outcome of a client's illness, that nurse will be prone to disappointment and frustration. However, if the nurse includes in her role responsibility to help the client achieve a peaceful death, both client and nurse will recognize their roles more precisely and be able to set realistic goals for themselves. Miss Henderson states: "the unique function of the nurse is to assist the individual, sick or well, in the performance of those activities contributing to health or its recovery (or to peaceful death) that he would perform unaided if he had the necessary strength, will, or knowledge."[17] The focus of nursing actions, according to Henderson, is to provide physical care for clients. The performance of these activities can be interpreted broadly to include intellectual, interpersonal, and technical activities. Miss Henderson's discussions of nursing and her illustrations of nursing functions suggest that she views nursing in this broad context.

A conscious awareness of one's personal philosophy and due consideration for human values, ethics, and beliefs are essential if one wants to develop his or her own definition of nursing. The following is the definition on which the content of this text is based: *Nursing is an encounter with a client and his family in which the nurse observes, supports, communicates, ministers, and teaches; she contributes to the maintenance of optimum health, and provides care during illness until the client is able to assume responsibility for the fulfillment of his own basic human needs; when necessary, she provides compassionate assistance with dying.*

The definition of nursing developed by each nurse may vary according to the language used, the setting one has in mind, and the personal orientation of the nurse according to her education and experience.

One can read any definition of nursing and assume or interpret the author's thoughts and intent. For example: the word *patient* can suggest that the author thinks of a person who is sick or not well and for whom she is responsible. This need not, but frequently does, exclude the preventive aspect of nursing. In the current decade, it would seem imperative that the nurse use the word *client* to express and show her concern for the prevention of illness as well as for the treatment needed for recovery.

The settings for nursing suggest that adaptability is necessary to cope with present situations. Today's journeys into space suggest that extraterrestrial nursing is a possibility; it can no longer be regarded as fictional. Until space stations are constructed, however, nursing needs on the planet earth are many and varied. The client who is the potential and actual recipient of nursing exists in a number of environs. Preventive and therapeutic nursing are needed in any setting; the intensity of the need varies with the degree or extent to which the service is needed, the point at which the client enters the health care system, and the place or setting in which he is thrust when the need for service arises.

Another variable in defining nursing is the breadth and depth of vision held by the nurse regarding the service she is able to provide. If her vision is myopic, she will provide a much different quality of service than the broad-visioned operator or agent. As one grows in maturity, in life, and in work experience, one sees him or herself and others more clearly, with more potential than when younger and less experienced. Each age has its merits, and a delicious blend of vigorous youth and healthy ripening or flowering maturity is a desirable mixture. Each learns from the other and benefits from open-minded exchanges to the ultimate benefit of the recipient of nursing—the client.

Despite variables in definitions of nursing, individual and groups of nurses should continue to strive to assemble words that represent their ideas and reflect the service of nursing as they see it. This would seem to be more important than continuing to look for one definition of nursing that will be universally accepted. Synonyms, in any language, allow for a number of words, any one, or any combination of which, can be used to describe the service nurses provide. A variety of resources should be used, including the potential of each concerned nurse to describe nursing; the definition of nursing should be expressed as a foundation for functioning. Then the nurse is ready to move to the essential actions of nursing, for which the definition is the springboard or beginning.

A review of nursing literature reveals that efforts have been made over the past 15 years to state a definition of nursing that can be accepted as universally as that given by Sister Olivia Gowan. Gradually, however, concern over a definition of nursing is being diluted by attempts to develop theoretic frameworks, develop theories that underlie nursing, define concepts inherent within nursing or that make nursing what it is—i.e., to clarify the art and science of nursing in the light of increasing knowledge in related biologic and behavioral fields of science.

More than a decade ago, nurses seemed to rely upon persons in related disciplines to show the way, point the direction, and define theories upon which nursing actions and roles could be based. Persons in the behavioral and physical science disciplines were generous in their assistance to the young profession, the fledgling group that had just begun to assume aspects of a profession. Results of an investigation, conducted under a research grant from the National Institute of Mental Health, prompted Johnson and Martin, two sociologists, to propose one type of theoretic base. They did not seek to answer all problems of nursing, but proposed a means by which nurses could view and analyze what they were doing. Beginning with the hypothesis that any social system has certain functional responsibilities, they defined these as: (a) making progress toward the defined goal or purpose for which the group exists; and (b) maintaining harmonious relationships among group members so that internal equilibrium can be maintained and the group will be cohesive and integrated. Actions to direct the group toward achieving its goals are called instrumental actions; actions for the purpose of maintaining equilibrium of group members are expressive actions.[18] This study focused primarily on the functioning of group members and secondly on the recipient of group action. This idea and framework can be applied to nursing in the following way: as members of the health team direct their efforts toward treating the client who is ill, their functions and actions are said to be *instrumental*. To achieve the desired goal of helping the client recover, communication among health team members, as well as collaboration and sharing plans, ideas, and efforts are necessary. The more effective the group is in maintaining a spirit of cooperation among its members, the more likely they are to achieve their goal of providing the client with the best care; these latter functions are termed *expressive* actions. Deliberate awareness of these differences in roles will assist in a more orderly and systematic analysis of nursing actions. The instrumental and expressive roles of the nurse are inherent in performing the nursing process.

Conceptualizing, theorizing, and intellectualizing are integral parts of nursing. Just as there has been a gradual but sure movement in nursing from performing actions instinctively, so has there been an effort to identify the intellectual aspect of nursing which directs the actions of the nurse. Also, efforts are being exerted to close the gap existing between the art and science of nursing, or the practice and intellectualizing of nursing. The goal of the science of nursing is defined as understanding, while that of the art of nursing is defined as skill, according to McKay. The art and science of nursing are integral parts of the nursing process. Science suggests knowledge, or intellectualization; art suggests action. "In the nursing process, both intelligence and technique are needed and, in addition, values must be upheld."[19]

CONCEPTS OF NURSING

In discussing the concept of nursing, the elements *concept* and *nursing* are difficult to define; a precise definition of each depends upon the intent of the person defining these elements.

One definition of a concept is: a mental impression, a general idea about the subject under consideration, the end-product of a thought process.

In each situation in nursing, a person performs an action for a receiver who needs some assistance. Nursing is the action, performed by a nurse, for a person with a particular need who is located in a particular setting. The action may be physical or mental; the person may involve a single individual, or one with a limited or a large family; the need may be potential or already existing; the setting may be a health agency or anywhere in the community. The following are examples:

THE ART	THE PERSON	THE NEED	THE SETTING
Caring for	*an acutely ill man*	*with a stroke*	*in the intensive care unit*
Helping	*a woman recovering from a stroke*	*with hemiplegia*	*in the rehabilitation unit*
Giving	*the employee*	*aspirin for a headache*	*in an industrial clinic*
Monitoring	*the astronauts*	*to keep them well*	*during space flight preparation*
Teaching	*a new mother*	*how to bathe her newborn*	*at home*
Caring	*for a soldier*	*with a bullet wound*	*on a battlefield*

Through a deliberate analysis of terms and their precise use, a more specific and clearer idea is conveyed to persons concerned about nursing.

A study was completed a few years ago in which the nursing literature was searched to determine what concepts existed.[20] Thirty concepts were found in two professional nursing periodicals in the 15-year period, 1950 to 1965. Twelve concepts appeared between the years 1950 and 1960. Eighteen concepts appeared in the years between 1960 and 1965. One of Horgan's assumptions was that concepts about nursing and the nursing process share components and elements in common. She defined a concept of nursing as: "an expression in words by the author of the ideas, which summarize the elements and components of what she thinks about nursing and the nursing process, or some aspect in this process." She concluded with the observation that nursing concepts were person- and action-centered; the persons were named by position—nurse and patient. Action was described as meeting patients' needs or as the nurse initiating a system or process to assess, fulfill, and validate the action necessary to meet patients' needs. Many of the concepts were not general; they were limited to specific stages or aspects of nursing or to a specific condition of the patient. The concepts did not emphasize the general health needs of people or nursing as a health service in society. The ultimate goals of nursing seemed to be meeting the needs of patients. Concepts seemed to center on the technology of assessing and validating needs, not on their fulfillment.

The need for sound theories and concepts to guide the practice of nursing has been expressed many times. Basic scientific theories can be accepted initially, tested, and evaluated as the nurse deliberately cares for clients. From the planned actions of practitioner, theories that guide her actions can be retested and reexplored, to assess their value and the extent to which they help to improve the practice of nursing. "Hunches" can be defined and ideas used to pursue further theories and actions, thereby setting up a continual cycle of activity—selecting a theory, using a theory to prescribe and plan nursing, testing the effectiveness of the action in terms of benefit to the client, revising, redefining, perhaps determining a new or selecting a different theory to use, testing and reevaluating for future actions. Hence, the deliberate use of theories assists in the sound planning and implementation of nursing actions, and results in qualitative nursing practice. Also, from sound nursing practice a body of theory will emerge that can be labeled the *theory of nursing*.

The theory of nursing is multifaceted and multidimensional. Just as there need not be just one definition of nursing because of the many variables operating, so there really are a number of theories that guide nursing action. Because the commodity provided in nursing is concerned with humans—the consumer is human, the agent or operator is human—there will be many definitions, concepts, and theories to guide nursing.

NURSING PROCESS

The term *nursing process* was not prevalent in the nursing literature until the mid-sixties; some limited evidence of the term appeared during the fifties. When the term was first introduced, the reaction of some nurses was: "We have been doing it all the time;" others said: "It is the same as the research process." It is true that nurses have followed the nursing process in the act of nursing; they have always determined the client's problems and planned how to cope with them. The effectiveness of the action was deliberately evaluated less often. The nurse uses the nursing process when she deliberately assesses the client's health problems, determines his and her role in coping with these problems, sets a plan of action which she is responsible for implementing, and then determines whether and how effective the action was.

In response to the statement: "it is the same as the research process," one can reply: "they are two different processes." "Purpose is the fundamental difference. The purpose of research is to reveal new knowledge; the purpose of problem solving is to solve an immediate problem in a particular setting."[21] Indeed, the solutions to certain problems can only be found through research; some problems may require new knowledge before they can be resolved. However, a large number of daily activities in nursing can be resolved by problem-solving techniques. The nursing process is essentially a problem-solving technique, but it also can be a useful tool in research.

On one occasion, in 1955, Lydia Hall spoke to a group of nurses in New Jersey about the quality of nursing care. Having once heard Mrs. Hall speak to a group, few could forget her unique platform style. The content of her presentation to the New Jersey group was unforgettable, too. She discussed her ideas about nursing, then stated the assumption basic to her total presentation: "Nursing is a process." She defined the use of four prepositions which indicate a relationship to and which can be used to describe the range in quality of the nursing process from not so good to very good. The four prepositions are: Nursing *at* the patient, *to* the patient, *for* the patient, and *with* the patient.[22]

Orlando's text was published at the beginning of the 1960s. For the past 10 years it has been referred to frequently for its presentation of the nursing process as well as for its differentiation of nursing activities. The central focus of Orlando's text, *The Dynamic Nurse-Patient Relationship*, was interpersonal relationship.[23] A proponent of deliberative actions, Orlando distinguished these from automatic activities that can become part of the nurse's functioning. She was as concerned for the client and his needs as were others who wrote about nursing. Orlando was one of the earliest authors to use the term, *the nursing process*. Although others had used the words, none had discussed the process in the same detail as did Orlando, nor had nurses been attracted to the label until the early years of the 1960s. Despite this "first," however, the term was not adopted immediately. Orlando identified a nursing situation as comprising three elements: (a) behavior of the patient, (b) reaction of the nurse, and (c) nursing actions designed for the patient's benefit. The interaction of these elements with each other is the nursing process.[23] Although attention was directed to the interpersonal aspect of care, appropriate attention to the physical and social aspects of care is included in the discussion of this concept. As did others who defined nursing and identified concepts of nursing, due attention is given to environmental influences as well as variables inherent in different settings in which nurses care for clients.

While Lydia Hall saw nursing as a process and Orlando defined phases of the process in terms of interpersonal relationships, other nurses were exploring ways of subdividing the process for analysis within a framework consistent with their philosophy and values.

In 1966, Lois Knowles presented a description of a model of the activities in which the nurse is engaged.[24] She suggested that the nurse's success as a practitioner depends on her mastery of the five D's; (a) Discover—she acquires knowledge or information about something that she did not know previously; such information should contribute to better client care. (b) Delve—she digs information from as many sources as possible to provide data about the client, which will assist her in providing for his care. (c) Decide—she plans the approach to use in the client's care. All facets of the problems are considered and the best course of action is designed. (d) Do—she administers, performs, and activates the plan that has been developed. (e) Discriminate—she distinguishes priorities and reactions by discerning differences in problems and the needs experienced by the client. Although not identical to phases of the nursing process as identified herein, these five D's suggest another way of approaching client care.[24]

In 1967, a committee involved with curriculum development in the Western States defined the nursing process as " . . . that which goes on between a patient and nurse in a given setting; it incorporates the behaviors of patient and nurse and the resulting interaction. The steps in the process are: perception, communication, interpretation, intervention, and evaluation."[25] Also, in 1967, a faculty group at the school of nursing at The Catholic University of American identified the phases of the nursing process as: assessing, planning, implementing, and evaluating.[26]

Few studies in nursing have been conducted in the same manner as the extensive research project that was undertaken by an interdiscipline group at the University of Colorado; the results were reported in a series of articles published in

Nursing Research over a period of years.[27-33] The purpose of the study was to investigate the clinical inference process as it referred to nursing. The responsibility of inferring the patient's needs was viewed as making judgments about the patient based on available data. Essentially, this can be interpreted as diagnosing the client's problems. When the client has particular problems, he will send out certain cues; the nurse is responsible for observing these. Through her observations of cues, she is able to make diagnoses, then decide on the best course of action to follow for the client's benefit.[28] These authors suggest that nurses have been engaged in this inferential process since nursing began but there has not been a critical, deliberate, and systematic analysis of the process until now. The *Lens Model* they suggest is easily adapted to the process of nursing. Significant landmarks in the model are: identification of the state of the patient from which cues are read or interpreted, inferences deduced, and the action planned and implemented according to defined goals. The authors illustrated the effectiveness of thorough analysis and the potential for study available in the fertile and complex nurse-client encounter.

To narrow the gap between the discovery of new knowledge and its application to the practice of nursing, Imogene King suggested that general concepts be identified; these then act as a broad base. As new knowledge is gained, the data acquired can be integrated into concepts already identified. Dr. King is to be saluted for making significant presentations of her own definition of nursing, defining and discussing concepts she feels are fundamental to its practice, and projecting their potential use in the development of a frame of reference that can be used for research in nursing practice. Nursing is defined by King as a process of action, reaction, interaction, and transaction whereby nurses assist individuals of any age group to meet their basic human needs in coping with their health status at some particular point in their life cycle. She suggests five concepts as a basis for organizing knowledge for nursing practice: Perception, communication, interpersonal relationships, health, and social institutions.[34]

At present, the term *nursing process* is accepted by nurses and it is viewed as the core process by which the purposes of nursing are fulfilled. In addition to nurses who developed concepts of the nursing process as a whole, others have contributed significantly to elements of the process, such as nursing history, nursing diagnosis, nursing orders, and nursing care plans.

Webster defines process as an action of moving forward, progressing from one point to another on the way to a goal, or to completion; it is the continuous movement through a succession of developmental stages; it is the method by which something is produced, something is accomplished, or a specific result is attained.[35]

To perceive a process as an action suggests a power behind the action or a mover of the action, hence control and/ or systematic movement. Conscious and deliberate effort must be exerted to arrive at a desired goal.

The absence of a planned or deliberate mover or movement results in a mechanical, automated effort, perhaps chaotic in nature, and certainly not orderly or systematic. Absence of a task or goal toward which a process is directed renders that process useless; it has no meaning if there is no purpose or potential for application. The basic concept of the process suggests it is a unified whole; it can be described in terms of phases, but each phase is dependent on the others— none stands alone. The elements can be distinguished for analysis and scrutiny, but for useful and practical purposes, a total concept of the process is necessary.

The nursing process is an orderly, systematic manner of determining the client's problems, making plans to solve them, initiating the plan or assigning others to implement it, and evaluating the extent to which the plan was effective in resolving the problems identified.

To use the nursing process in the desired manner, each nurse must develop certain behaviors so that her efforts will be more effective and the client will receive better care. Her innate abilities and acquired knowledge will be fundamental to any nursing performance. The interpersonal techniques one learns throughout life enable the nurse to know herself and to deal with others. Dealing effectively with others pre-

sents a continuing challenge that usually motivates and stim-
ulates the nurse to think in terms of coping with each individual. To achieve qualitative results, nursing behavior
should include problem-solving orientation, and problem-
solving techniques should be developed deliberately.[36]

Certain behaviors will prove more successful than others
in helping the nurse use her abilities and knowledge. Creativity, adaptability, commitment, trust, and leadership are
characteristics or behaviors conducive to the better performance of nursing actions that comprise the nursing process.

The creative nurse initiates change; she sees potential development and continued improvement of actions. She is able
to pursue goals and perform necessary intellectual, interpersonal, and technical procedures and techniques for effective client care, yet she is looking beyond immediate activities to find better ways to accomplish the same goals. She
need not be an activist or a rebel, but she needs vision and
insight so that she does not become embedded in a rut from
which she may find it difficult to dislodge herself.

Adaptability suggests that the nurse is able to move with
whatever situation she encounters; she is able to adjust to
varying demands of the same or several situations; she is able
to employ acceptable and appropriate means to provide care
for various clients with different backgrounds and individual
idiosyncrasies. This suggests that she has a plan; she does not
enter the situation unprepared; rather she validates her perceptions with the client and plans with him, adjusting and
changing this plan where necessary. Adaptability suggests
flexibility with enough structure to promote the process of
nursing.

The successful nurse is the committed nurse. She is the
person who sees the client as an individual; respects him for
his person and his humanity; and respects his rights, his beliefs, and his interest in himself. Concern for herself is a part
of the committed nurse's interest; however, this self-concern
is intended to promote more careful assessment of herself so
that she can become more aware of her own abilities and
limitations, thus making her more capable of dealing with

client concerns and needs. There is a good portion of selfless-ness inherent in the committted nurse's actions.

To cope with the care of any client, there must be mutual trust. Only when the client feels that the nurse trusts him will he be able to share needed information with her. Any sense of distrust will destroy this relationship, once it has been established, or any potential relationship. Just as the client must be able to trust the nurse, so the nurse must be able to trust the client. Honesty in dealing with each other will en-courage this mutual trust relationship and once established, it will be a solid foundation on which to build future and fur-ther encounters.

Leadership in pursuit of the nursing process is a desirable trait. Personal abilities and healthy initiative foster the de-velopment of a model of desirable behavior, which is needed to pursue the nursing process. With capable leader-ship qualities, the nurse initiates changes, uses creativity, and performs as a role model to promote a sense of trust, a feeling of commitment, and to utilize adaptability in an effective way.

Dividing the process into phases is an artificial separation of actions, which, in actual practice, cannot be separated. To insure a deliberateness and thoughtfulness in proceeding through the process, however, it is necessary to label the phases and suggest that the practitioner make a concerted effort to name each action in terms of the phase of nursing she is performing. This practice will insure that the *how* of the nursing process and the *how* of nursing action are care-fully, consciously, and deliberately pursued. The *what* of nursing will not be as uniformly labeled as the *how* of nursing, for the *what* will vary with each client. To facilitate the discussion and performance of nursing, the nursing pro-cess is divided into the following components or phases: as-sessing, planning, implementing, and evaluating. Although other authors use similar names for each phase of the process, it is believed that these four labels best identify the phases through which nursing proceeds. Each phase of the nursing process will be defined and the components of each phase will be identified so as to introduce theories basic to the nursing process, as presented in Chapter 2. (An in-depth analysis and discussion of each of the four phases of the nursing process will be presented in Chapter 3.)

Assessing

Assessing is the act of reviewing a situation for the purpose of diagnosing the client's problems.

So that the nurse can judge which actions are necessary to assist the client with his problems, she uses her skills of perception, observation, and communication.

Perception suggests insight into various facets of a situation. The nurse develops insight into what she is seeing as a client's problem, insight into what she is hearing the client say he needs, and insight into how these data relate to each other. The nurse reflects on similar situations she has encountered in the past, on the significance and meaning of various cues she is perceiving, and on the variety of human factors she is able to identify in the situation. Foresight is necessary too. While the nurse observes the client's immediate status, she will also be thinking of his future. For example: an instrument maker who enters the emergency room with a relatively serious injury to his thumb will have immediate needs; with her immediate actions, the nurse simultaneously thinks of the questions that will arise: Will job adjustment be necessary? How soon will prognosis be known? What can he be told if he asks about prognosis?

The art of communication includes talking as well as listening. Communication with the client begins with the first face-to-face contact between him and the nurse. A deliberately worded greeting and listening carefully to the client's reply will set the stage for a good encounter.

Utilizing a predetermined format on which to record information about the client insures that data helpful to nursing personnel as they plan his care will be collected; also, by recording the information the client will not have to repeat it to a number of different personnel. This implies the need for pertinent information to be communicated to all nursing team personnel collaborating in the client's care. Various nursing history forms have been developed and used by nurses to insure that data about the client are collected; several have been reported in the literature.[37, 38] The exact form can be developed from those that have been published, or nurses can develop an original form that will best meet the requirements of a particular situation. It is not important that nurses everywhere use the same type of form; it is important, however, that a format be used as an organized method of obtaining data about the client.

For a number of years, *diagnosis* was a charged and forbidden word in nursing. A literal definition of the word, with no qualifier preceding it, suggests it is a good word to use when conveying the idea that one is seeking knowledge or information about what needs to be corrected, or what it is that is causing some difficulty, or what is interfering with normal functions. With this idea in mind, nursing can use the word diagnosis as effectively as can the physician, or any person who is trying to discover where his efforts must be applied to perform his service for the benefit of his client or customer. The difference lies in the purpose of the diagnosis. The goal of a nursing diagnosis is different from that of a medical diagnosis; the physician is concerned with diagnosing the cause of illness so that he can treat the underlying pathologic process. He obtains a medical history, asking significant questions, using observation, collecting data from the client which he will analyze and about which he will draw conclusions so that he can plan the patient's medical and therapeutic regimen.[39] The nurse essentially follows the same process, examining, asking questions, and observing, but her efforts are directed toward diagnosing the client's presenting symptoms.[27] She will be interested in the conclusions drawn by the physician in his exploration, since she will be assisting with the therapeutic plan. Her diagnosis of the client will be different from that determined by the physician. For example: the medical diagnosis of a client who has suffered a stroke may include: cerebrovascular accident, arteriosclerosis, and diabetes mellitus. The nursing diagnosis may include:

dysphagia, hemiplegia (right), mentally alert, and aphasia. Nursing diagnoses provide the basis for nursing orders, which are prescriptions the nurse considers essential for the client's welfare. Nursing orders are communicated among the nursing staff and are revised as necessary, according to nursing diagnoses. Nursing and medical diagnoses, along with nursing and medical orders, comprise the therapeutic plan for the client; the orders complement each other and the client is the beneficiary of collaborative efforts in planning his care based on nursing and medical diagnoses.

Planning

Planning means to determine what can be done to assist the client; it involves setting goals, judging priorities, and designing methods to resolve problems.

Judicious, careful, and deliberate goal-setting is vital to this phase of the nursing process so that the nursing care plan can be developed. When goals are defined, the blueprint is drawn, and methods are identified as to the best way to accomplish established goals.

Having collected pertinent data about the client through assessment, the nurse continues to validate these data. By communicating with the client to determine whether her perceptions are correct, the nurse will insure that she and the client are at the same point in the planning phase and that both have assessed and perceived his problems in the same way. Long-range or ultimate goals, as well as short-range or proximate goals, will be established, within which priorities are set. The most urgent or the one that should be achieved first is determined before long-range or more distant goals are set. Proximate goals can be likened to wayside stations, in that they can be attained more quickly; they give both the client and nurse some degree of satisfaction as well as a sense of accomplishment and some assurance that steps toward the ultimate goal are well directed. Both goals are kept in sight, and the actions needed to achieve both ultimate and proximate goals proceed simultaneously, but each is at a different stage of development.

The essence of planning includes a deliberate approach to setting precise goals, both ultimate and proximate, continually validating the data obtained by assessing the client's problems, establishing priorities, and making decisions about specific measures to be used to resolve his problems.

By assessing the client's problems deliberately and systematically through knowledgeable perception, observation, and communication, validating her findings rather than relying on her intuition, the nurse provides qualitative data from which accurate diagnoses can be made and sound planning developed.[40]

Implementation

Implementation involves action; it is the phase in which the nurse initiates and completes the actions necessary to accomplish defined goals.

Thought and preparation were involved in assessing and planning, and decisions were made about actions required to help the client. As she implements these actions, the nurse will be coordinating the activities of various paramedical personnel and functioning cooperatively with a number of people on the health scene for the benefit of the client. The exact number of these persons will vary, depending upon the setting in which the client is located. Caring for a client at home will involve different kinds of personnel than, for example, caring for that same client in a medical center in which teaching and research are emphasized. In either setting, the nurse will be coping with people who will be interrupting actions, seeking data about the client, and invading the territory of nurse and client, but all of these people will be a vital part of the health scene.

Personnel from various disciplines, functioning on the health team, are acting on behalf of the client; the mere presence of a number of people in the client's environment means that their activities must be coordinated to make sure that all are directed toward his best interests. Most of the responsibility for coordinating these actions belongs to the nurse. This implies good interpersonal relations and a knowledge of human behavior. Coordinating the various activities successfully so that defined goals are achieved through the action of various people is a challenging task and one that can act as a major motivating force for the professional nurse.

Within the nursing team there are levels of personnel with different kinds of preparation as well as different personality traits and abilities. The nurse assumes responsibilities for direct client care and for coordinating the efforts of and directing the activities of nursing team personnel. Involved in this responsibility is the need for knowing the potential production level of each member of the nursing team, knowing the problems and needs of the clients for whom they are responsible, and matching these two quantities to the best of her ability. This is a constant task, a dynamic activity, to which the committed nurse can address herself with qualitative results. The skillful application of techniques of interpersonal relations can bring about positive and pleasing outcomes for the client as well as satisfaction for personnel.

Implementation is an action-oriented phase of the nursing process in which the nurse is responsible for implementing the nursing care plan that was developed. To be able to coordinate skillfully the activities of health and nursing team members, minister direct client care, and delegate responsibilities for this care to nursing personnel, according to their backgrounds and abilities, are challenges confronting the nurse during this phase. The intellectual, interpersonal, and technical actions employed during the implementation phase are based on the plan for nursing care designed for the individual client according to his assessed problems.

Evaluation

Evaluation means to appraise the client's behavioral changes due to the actions of the nurse.

To initiate the evaluation phase, the nurse must review and reflect on the goals set by the original blueprint or nursing care plan devised for the client. When goals are established, and aims identified at the outset of client care, the nurse and client are able to determine whether, and to what extent, they have reached their destination. This process of determining just where they are in goal-attainment will involve asking a number of questions. The nurse will be concerned with: What were the expected client behaviors? Is there another way of moving, or acting, to accomplish the same goals with more efficiency or more effectiveness for the client? What changes should, or could, be made? Did the nurse achieve the goals she set out to accomplish? Should some adjustments be made so that these same actions can be more effective? Planning for future actions for this and other clients will be adjusted or altered by this type of constant evaluation and inquiry.

The nursing audit is a form of evaluation that has a great deal of potential for improving client care. Auditing the developed nursing care plans presents a type of reflective evaluation before actual care is administered. These plans can be reviewed for completeness, thoroughness, and for the use of good judgment, according to the types of problems the client experienced. Actual client care can be audited by a systematic plan devised by nurses who minister to the clients. The legal record contains an after-the-fact documentation of the care performed; these records also can be audited. Auditing legal records is the one facet of the nursing audit that has been developed best in the literature;[41] however, the entire nursing audit is a fertile area of evaluation for nurses to explore and develop.

Evaluation involves a reflecting or looking back at the actions taken to determine how effective these were in terms of client behavioral changes. This has been a neglected phase of the nursing process, perhaps because there is a paucity of tools whereby the nurse could evaluate her actions with a high degree of objectivity. Some subjectivity enters into any human evaluation, but nurses are constantly striving to minimize it. Until more precise methods become available for measuring the extent to which goals have been achieved, the evaluation phase of the nursing process will continue to need further attention and development.

SUMMARY

The profession of nursing has moved through a number of stages that can be relatively well defined by reflecting on the progress of nursing through the years. From debating about whether or not nursing is a profession, the group has moved to the more serious concern of defining the essence of nursing. A number of nurse authors have suggested ideas and definitions that identify the unique nature of nursing according to individual orientations and philosophies. Concepts of nursing are being identified with increasing frequency, and more precise and qualifying theories are emerging. Eventually, the science of nursing will be clearly labeled. Finally, the nursing process has been accepted as the very core of nursing, and although there are several ways in which each of the phases or components of the process are labeled, the idea of the process is well accepted and the steps through which the nurse proceeds to effect client care have the general support of nursing.

REFERENCES

1. Frank C M: Foundations of Nursing. Philadelphia, W B Saunders Co, 1959, p 78
2. Nightingale F: Notes on Nursing. What It Is and What It Is Not. (facsimile of 1859 edition). Philadelphia, J B Lippincott Co, 1946
3. Brown E L: Nursing For the Future. New York, Russell Sage Foundation, 1948
4. Flexner A: Universities. New York, Oxford University Press, 1930
5. Schein, E H: Professional Education—Some New Directions. New York, McGraw-Hill Book Co, 1972, pp 7-14
6. Coladarci A P: What about that word profession? Am J Nurs 63:116-118
7. American Nurses' Association. Code for Nurses. Am J Nurs 68:2581-2585
8. American Nurses' Association's First Position on Education For Nursing. Am J Nurs 65:106-111
9. Toward Quality in Nursing. Needs and Goals. Report of the Surgeon General's Consultant Group on Nursing. US Department of Health, Education, and Welfare, Public Health Service, 1963

10. Lysaught J P: An Abstract For Action. New York, McGraw-Hill Book Co, 1970, pp 81-147
11. Gowan S M O: Administration of college and university programs in nursing, from the viewpoint of nurse education. Proceedings of the Workshop on Administration of College Programs in Nursing. Washington, DC, The Catholic University of America Press, 1944, p 10
12. Kreuter F: What is good nursing care? Nurs Outlook 57:302-304
13. Erikson E H: Childhood and Society. Second edition. New York, W W Norton and Co, Inc, 1963, pp 247-251
14. Johnson D E: A philosophy of nursing. Nurs Outlook 7:198-200, 1959, p 199, 200
15. *Idem:* The nature of a science of nursing. Nurs Outlook 7:291-294, 1959
16. Weidenbach E: The helping art of nursing. Am J Nurs 63:54-57
17. Henderson V: The Nature of Nursing. New York, The Macmillan Company, 1966, p 15
18. Johnson M M, Martin H W: A sociological analysis of the nurse role. Am J Nurs 58:373-377
19. McKay R P: The Process of Theory Development in Nursing. New York, Teachers College, Columbia University, A Report of an Ed D Project, 1965, p 16
20. Horgan S M Visitation: Concepts About Nursing in Selected Nursing Literature from 1950-1965. Unpublished Masters Dissertation, The Catholic University of America, School of Nursing, 1967
21. Wandelt M A: Guide for the Beginning Researcher. New York, Appleton-Century-Crofts, 1970
22. Hall L E: Quality of Nursing Care. Address at meeting of Department of Baccalaureate and Higher Degree Programs of the New Jersey League for Nursing, February 7, 1955, Seton Hall University, Newark, New Jersey. Published in Public Health News, New Jersey State Department of Health, June, 1955
23. Orlando I J: The Dynamic Nurse-Patient Relationship. New York, G P Putman's Sons, 1961, p 26
24. Knowles L N: Decision making in nursing—a necessity for doing, ANA Clinical Sessions, 1966. New York, Appelton-Century-Crofts, 1967, pp 248-272
25. Western Interstate Commission on Higher Education, 1967, p 6. Defining Clinical Content, Graduate Nursing Programs, Medical and Surgical Nursing.
26. The Nursing Process. Edited by H Yura, M Walsh. Washington, D C, The Catholic University of America Press, 1967
27. Kelly K J: An approach to study of clinical inference in nursing. Nursing Res 13:314-322, 1964
28. *Idem:* Clinical inference in nursing—a nurse's viewpoint. Nurs Res 15:23-26, 1966
29. *Idem:* Clinical inference in nursing—a psychologist's viewpoint. Nurs Res 15:27-38, 1966

30. Hammond K R, Kelly, K J, Castellan, N J Jr, Schneider, R J: Clinical inference in nursing—analyzing cognitive tasks representative of nursing problems. Nurs Res 15:134-138, 1966

31. *Idem:* Clinical inference in nursing—information units used. Nurs Res 15:236-243, 1966

32. Hammond K R, Kelly K J, Castellan N J Jr, Schneider R J, Vancini M: Clinical inference in nursing: use of information seeking strategies. Nurs Res 15:330-336, 1966

33. *Idem:* Clinical inference in nursing—revising judgments. Nurs Res 16:38-45, 1967

34. King I: A conceptual frame of reference for nursing. Nurs Res 17:27-31, 1968

35. Webster's Third International Dictionary. Massachusetts, G and C Merriam Co, 1967

36. McDonald F J, Harms T: A theoretical model for an experimental curriculum, Nurs Outlook 14:48-50, 1966

37. McPhetridge L M: Nursing History: One means to personalized care. Am J Nurs 68:68-75, 1968

38. Smith D: A Clinical Nursing tool. Am J Nurs 68:2384-2388, 1968

39. Carlson S: A practical approach to the nursing process. Am J Nurs 72:1589-1591, 1972

40. McCain F: Nursing by assessment, not intuition. Am J Nurs 65:82-85, 1965

41. Phaneuf M: The Nursing Audit. New York, Appleton-Century-Crofts, 1972

chapter two

Theoretic Framework

The nursing process is a designated series of actions intended to fulfill the purposes of nursing—maintain the client's wellness and, if this state changes, provide the amount and quality of nursing care his situation demands to direct him back to wellness, and if wellness cannot be achieved, to contribute to his quality of life, maximizing his resources as long as life is a reality. To fulfill these purposes, the development of the idea of the nursing process and the beginning development of its theoretic framework must be considered.

Many different theories from various disciplines suggest a relationship to the nursing process. These include general systems theory, information theory, communication theory, decision theory, and theories of perception. General systems theory seems to be applicable in a broad way. Theories from information, communication, and decision stem from that of the general systems and give support in a more specific manner. Selections from these theories give credence to the nurse's as well as the client's actions and provide a framework within which the nursing process can be analyzed and applied.

GENERAL SYSTEMS THEORY

General systems theory provides a framework for dealing with complex problems and their changing relationships. A system can be viewed as an entity composed of interrelated interacting parts or components. A system is comprised of purpose, process, and content. Purpose refers to that which must be accomplished and therefore gives direction to the system; content refers to the parts that make up the system, while the process of the system and its operations are functions of the parts in fulfilling the purpose for which the system was developed. Banathy states that the best way to identify a system is to reveal its purpose.[1]

General systems theory was introduced by Ludwig von Bertalanffy when it appeared that there were laws within this system that applied to all systems of a certain type, irrespective of their particular properties and the elements involved. Thus, von Bertalanffy postulated a general system theory whose subject matter is the formulation of principles valid for all systems, regardless of the nature of or the relationship between their component elements. The aim of general systems theory is to integrate the various fields of science with unifying principles that extend vertically through each individual science.[2] Thus, communication between specialists from different disciplines could be enhanced, and the duplication of effort resulting from identical formulations developed independently, could be eliminated. General systems theory provides the structure through which a whole may be broken into its component parts so that the relationship or force between them can be studied and manipulated. It also provides a structure whereby unconnected parts may be integrated into an organized whole.

A system may be composed of subsystems, each designed to carry out a purpose, which, in turn, is necessary in achieving the general purpose of the system. Nursing operates within the context of the health care system and, as such, may be considered one of its subsystems. The health care system is not an enclosed self-sustaining one but operates within the environment that gives it its purpose. Society can be considered the suprasystem of the health care system, for the former gives the latter its purpose. Thus, the health care system has its own purpose, process, and content, as well as its own resources, demands, and limitations. Many other systems operate within the suprasystem of society—educational, political, industrial. The health care system operates cooperatively in conjunction with these other systems. Within the health care system there are a number of subsystems designed to carry out the purpose of the health care system. Nursing, medicine, dentistry, and pharmacy are but a few of such subsystems. Each carries out a specific purpose which, in turn, contributes to attaining that of the health care system. Subsystems which operate in an integrated cooperative manner contribute to the effectiveness of the health care system, thus fulfilling the purpose for which it exists, as designated by society. The health care system derives input from the suprasystem—society. Through interacting components (functioning within their purposes, input, resources as derived from the suprasystem), output is produced and fed back into the suprasystem. The closer the output satisfies the purpose for which the system exists, the more acceptable the output will be to the suprasystem. Society will reject output that does not fulfill its purpose. Therefore, the system's output must be assessed continually to make sure that it is adequate. Effective feedback from the suprasystem is needed to maintain its compatibility and viability. Implied in this is a sensitivity to the changing needs and purposes of society and a willingness to make appropriate adjustments. The system will need to look into itself for ways of maximizing the interaction of its components, as well as to assess the effectiveness with which each subsystem within the health care system is performing.[1] The diagram in Figure 1 incorporates the system idea.

With nursing considered a subsystem of the health care system, general systems theory can provide a useful framework for the study of nursing. The concepts and principles of general systems theory offer a decision-making structure as well as a set of strategies which could be used to arrive at a decision. These comprise a self-correcting logical process for assessing, planning, implementing, and evaluating a plan of

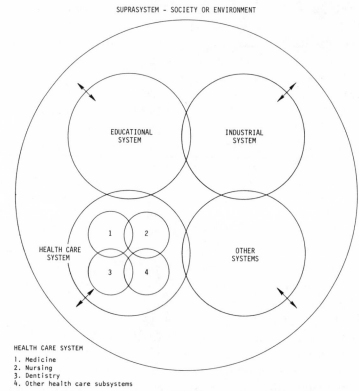

FIG. 1.

action to fulfill the purposes of nursing. Basically, this is a practical application of the problem-solving method. Figure 2 demonstrates the elements of the nursing subsystem—the nurse and the client. The elements of the system are interacting. Nurse and client are each unique in that they have different behavior systems. Thus, the dynamic interaction between her behavior and that of the person or persons who are the client(s) constitute a complex organized whole. The nursing process, with its components—assessing, planning, implementing, and evaluating—constitutes a unifying process utilized to fulfill the purposes of nursing. Through the nursing process information is processed, problems are designated, alternatives for action are delineated, and a selection is made for implementation. Evaluation is built into the process, with reassessment and modification important aspects

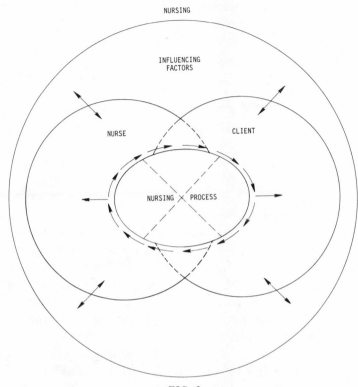

FIG. 2.

to insure the purposefulness of acts directed toward a specified goal. Influencing factors related to nursing and which
have an impact on elements of the system include: role designations, role expectations, educational preparation and level,
place of interaction, history and tradition, trends, economy,
values, transportation, availability of health services.

The concepts of general systems theory are open systems,
closed systems, energy and matter, entropy, negentropy, information, and feedback. Systems may be closed or open. A
closed system is considered isolated from its environment in
that neither matter, energy, nor information are exchanged
with it. Laws of thermodynamics focus only on closed systems. In these systems a certain quantity must increase to a
maximum and the process eventually stops in a state of equilibrium. This certain quantity is called entropy, and in a

closed system the tendency is toward maximum entropy or disorder. Thus, a system is closed if no material leaves or enters it.

The open system is one in which there is an exchange of matter, energy, or information with the environment. A person is viewed as a living behaving system. The nurse and the client can each be studied as persons. For example, let us consider the biochemical, psychosocial, value, and attitudinal systems of each person. Each of these systems are subsystems; each has its own purpose which, in turn, contribute to the functioning of a person as a whole as well as the goals of that person. In nursing, the nurse and client interact in a dynamic fashion for a purpose.

An open system maintains itself in a continuous inflow and outflow, building up its components and breaking them down, but never reaching a state of equilibrium. The open system maintains itself in a steady state. The composition of the system remains constant despite the fact that energy, matter, or information are imported and exported; the process is one of building up and breaking down, in spite of continuous irreversible processes. There are remarkable regulatory characteristics evident in the steady state. This steadiness is referred to as the principle of equifinality. A steady state can be reached from different initial conditions and after disturbances develop in the process.[2] A living system can avoid an increase in entropy and develop toward a state of increased order and organization.[3] An example of this type of exchange is the temperature regulating system of the body,[4] wherein the body increases the amount of heat it produces when it enters a cool environment. Shivering is one method whereby the body increases its heat production and the person may follow through by putting on more clothing or turning up the thermostat. A hot environment induces a response designed to cool the body—sweating. The evaporation of moisture on the surface of the skin has a cooling effect. Additional measures might include removing some clothing, lowering the temperature setting of a thermostat, or turning on an air conditioner. The metabolic, the growth, and the total processes of living and being involve the interchange of energy, matter, or information among parts of the living organism and between the living organism and its environment. That energy or information taken in or absorbed is called input; the energy, matter, or information that passes out of the organism into the environment is called output.[5] When viewed as a behaving system alone, man is quite simple. However, the complex environment in which man exists is reflected in the obvious complexity of man's behavior as it develops with age. Hazzard points out that the living organism is an excellent example of a system, because it comprises many interrelated elements and is capable of developing toward states of increased order, organization, differentiation, or disintegration.[4]

Energy and matter are concepts of general systems theory. Energy, in a physical sense, means the capacity to do work and overcome resistance. Matter may be defined as a space-occupying mass—the substance that can be exchanged.

Entropy can be used as an indication of the state of health of a living system. Raymond believes that life processes that are disturbed because matter or energy is poorly transmitted through the organism may, at times, be viewed in terms of deficiencies in information for the direction of required reactions. As the structural and behavioral information content of various parts of the body are destroyed, entropy increases as the living system proceeds toward death. The degenerative processes of nature balance out when the steady state is maintained by fuels that have a high free-energy content and by communicated information. In the person, communication is carried on through the nervous system, by the transmission of pressure through the vascular system, and through the production and transport of hormones and enzymes. The living system needs sufficient information to facilitate rapid adjustment to a wide variety of information inputs so that growth and adaptability will be enhanced.[6] The human organism's struggle to grow and to develop is accomplished by a continual interchange of matter, energy, or information between it and the environment. The goal is a steady state, maximizing negative entropy as the human organism tends toward order.

The nurse and the client are regarded as a system that has a certain repertoire of internal and external basic acts, various combinations and sequences of which make up its behaviors. The client may be an individual or a family. A family fulfills the criteria of a system because it consists of interrelated parts that are capable of reacting to changes in the environment in its efforts to maintain a steady state. If the behavior of the human organism is to adapt to its environment, the selective process by which its basic acts are linked together must be organized according to the current status of the environment relative to the organism.[7]

The ideas of information and feedback provide a frame of reference for viewing a wide range of situations. The person is viewed as a living, behaving system and as an open system engaged in dynamic interchange with his environment. He is self-organizing, adaptive, self-aware, goal-seeking, and learns. He needs information and depends on the process of communication between and/or among systems as well as subsystems and their environments.[8] Information is defined as some type of event in the physical world which will permit movement over space.[9] Rapaport defines a quantity of information as a signal selected from a set or matched with an element of a set.[10]

Information in the context of general systems theory is measured in terms of decisions and selective process. Information is similar to negative entropy, which is a measure of order. The concept of information is viewed as a tool for quantifying data; that of entropy and negative entropy or negentropy refers to the measure of order and disorder in a system. Entropy is recognized as a measure of disorder. Schrödinger states that every happening, event, and process going on in nature means that in that part of the world where they are going on entropy has increased. A living organism continually increases its entropy, tending to approach the dangerous state of maximum entropy—death. Feeding upon negative entropy by eating, breathing, drinking, and assimilating, the living organism avoids death.[11]

Feedback is a process whereby information about output from a system is communicated back to that system so that it can be evaluated and regulated. It constitutes the control mechanism of the system, relating output back to its source so that it is possible to make adjustments, adaptations, and modifications. Feedback is an extremely important component, if the system is to regulate itself. The evaluation component of the nursing process incorporates feedback in designating problem-solution or need for reassessment.

INFORMATION AND COMMUNICATION THEORY

In addition to the theoretic framework provided by general systems theory in a broad sense, additional theoretic formulations relating to information and communication, decisions, and perception shed more insight into the basis for these processes. These theories have contributed to systems theory. A cardinal feature of information theory is that it is a theory of selection—selection from well-defined sets of alternatives. To make a selection is to make a decision. Such a theory is statistical in the sense that probability must be considered.[10] The wider the choice, the larger the set of alternatives open to use. The more uncertain one is about how to proceed, the more information that person requires before he can make a decision. Involved in efficient communication is the analysis of how a person selects and codes available stimuli, that is, how effectively does he process his input. Information and communication theory focus on the fundamental nature of the mediating linkage underlying the interrelations and interactions of the parts that comprise a complex living, behaving system. A person needs information when confronted with some sort of choice to make. Information processes, being selective, demand that selections be made from a set of alternatives. If the sequence of selection is to convey information, the possible choice must be known to the person who is to receive that information. It is necessary to consider the choices available to us and the probabilities associated with each.[12] The information transmitted depends on the manner in which and how effectively sensory input from the environment is processed and organized. Information is the number of potential choices provided from which effective courses of action can be selected. Ackoff states that to inform is to provide a basis for choice—a belief in the greater efficiency of one choice over another. He believes information modifies the objective probabilities of choice by modifying subjective estimates of probabilities of success. Instruction is seen as modifying the probabilities of success. Further, a person's state of instruction can be characterized by the amount of control he can exercise over the outcomes within his sphere of responsibility. The more capable a person is in bringing about any of the outcomes possible, the greater control he has over that outcome. This capability can be acquired through instruction.[13]

Communication focuses on the essential nature of the mediating connection underlying the interrelations and interactions within and between systems. The concept of meaning enters into communication because both the sender and receiver must know what a given set of symbols signifies. The components of a communication system are: source, transmitter, channel, receiver, destination. The source formulates meaning into a message while the transmitter encodes or transforms that message into information. The source and transmitter are different phases of the act of communication initiated by the person who originated or sent the message. The channel for transmission may be the atmosphere, in the case of a verbal message, or, if it is written, telegraphic or other means are used to carry the information from one area to another.[9] The receiver decodes the information by transforming its physical aspects into a message. Transformation into the final component, "destination," whose function is to interpret the meaning of the message, is accomplished by a person's perceptual abilities. Communication takes place if its meaning at the source of origin coincides with that at its destination. Perfect correspondence between denotative and connotative responses of source and destination is seldom achieved due to interference, which may be mechanical, psychologic, or cultural. This interference, from whatever cause, is called *noise* and needs to be recognized as an additional component of the theoretic system of the act of communication. Correspondence between elements of the response pattern, constituting the meaning at the source and its counterpart at the destination, is reduced, to some degree, by noise. Another factor in the act of communicating is feedback. The destination operates as a source of feedback, which constitutes a kind of message returning to the communicator. This feedback may take the form of nonverbal communication, and as such can be affected by noise in that gestures or facial expressions can be misunderstood. Thus, this two-way set of components operates as a communication system, with information moving first one way and then another, or both ways at the same time.[9] This is especially true for person-to-person communication within a system or with persons in other systems. Verbal messages are not the only source of information. A person also may obtain information by observation.

In Mackay's informational analysis of responses to questions, he states that a question is basically a purported indication of inadequacy as to the state of readiness of its originator and is calculated to elicit some organizing work to remedy his inadequacy. It would seem that the questioner uncovers and holds out the incomplete portion of his organizing system to the person receiving his attention. Mackay points out that the primary purpose of a question is to update the questioner's own state of readiness. In turn, the meaning of the answer will be its selective function on the range of the questioner's state of orientation.[7]

Ackoff's conceptualization of information relates to the problems the recipient has in reaching a decision. He acknowledges behavioral elements in purposeful states as an individual's objectives, his valuation of each objective, his possible course of action, the efficiency of each course of action in achieving each objective, and his probability of choice for each course of action. The amount of information in a purposeful state is seen in terms of the probabilities of choices for available courses of action, while the amount of information in a message is the difference between that following and that preceding the message. Motivation relates to the values the person has placed on the objectives.[13] Communication that changes the probabilities of choice, informs. If changes in the efficiencies of courses of action are noted, the communication is one that instructs. When the values of outcome are changed, communication motivates. A single communication may combine information with instruction and motivation.[13] It must be remembered that an inner environment of the living system places limits on the kind of information-processing of which the organism is capable. The inner environment imposes very broad limits on organization. Limits are imposed not only on language but also on every other mode of communication, representing, internally, the experiences received through stimuli from outside.[5]

The conceptual framework of information and communication theory can serve as a basis for decision theory, which is seen as the selection and application of a criterion that should be used in selecting a course of action, a purposeful state. Decision theory concerns itself with efficiency, value, and effectiveness.

The purpose of nursing is to identify the client's problems, whether he is well or ill. The nursing process, as the significant process used by the nurse, is basically a decision process. The deliberate use of the nursing process demands that the nurse have knowledge. It involves seeking, selecting, and processing information, judging that information, designating priorities about the information, awareness of alternatives and choosing them, as well as implementing a formulated plan of action. Continuous feedback or evaluation requires appropriate modification of the plan of action to maintain its purposefulness. Keen perception, communication, and effective decisions are inherent in this process. The nursing process is cyclic because the need for modification demands reassessment, replanning, renewed implementation, and reevaluation.

DECISION THEORY

One goal in the deliberative use of the nursing process is to solve a problem. The nursing process can be used to design a course of action aimed at changing an existing situation into a preferred one. Solving a problem means to represent it in such a manner that its solution becomes transparent.[5] The more difficult and novel the problem is, the more likely trial and error will be required to find a solution. Trial and error are highly selective and represent progress toward a goal. Indications of progress spur further search in the same direction while a lack of progress is a signal to look elsewhere for the solution. This is another way of demonstrating the cyclic nature of the nursing process with its built-in evaluation component, determining progress toward a goal. If the goal is not reached, the course of action must be modified and reassessed. Problem-solving requires selective trial and error. A decision is made as to which path to try first and what data are promising.[5] Simon states that when we examine sources from which the problem-solving system derives its selectivity, that selectivity can always be equated with some kind of information feedback from the environment. There are basically two kinds of selectivity: (a) various paths are tried, consequences noted, and this information used as a guide to further search, and (b) previous experience. When a problem to be solved is comparable to one resolved previously, similar paths may again be tried. Given a desired and an existing state, the task of an adaptive organism is to find the difference between these two states and the correlating process that would erase the difference. The task is to discover a sequence of processes that would produce the desired goal from the initial state. The activity of human problem-solving is a form of means-to-an-end analysis aimed at discovering a process description of the path that leads to a desired goal.[5] The nursing process is such a process. The primacy of goal-attainment, as a function of a system, gives priority to processes involved most directly with the success or failure of goal-oriented endeavors.

Inherent in problem-solving activity are choices, decisions about choices, and decisions about decisions. Daniel Griffiths[14] analyzes the decision-making process and contends that all decision-makers operate within a set of limits, thereby improving the caliber of the decisions they make. Preparation for a particular decision begins in the past of the person who is making that decision—before the first formal step is taken in the process. Initially, the problem must become known before the decision-maker can go about defining the problem. This is accomplished when the nurse attempts to state the problems either in terms of her goals or those of a client. The problem is stated in such a way that the decision-maker can grasp its significance.

Within the limitations defined by purpose, the criterion of rationality, conditions of employment, lines of formal authority, relevant information provided, and time limits, how to arrive at a decision as well as the content of that decision can be prescribed.[14] The following steps comprise the decision-making process:

1. Recognize, define, and limit the problem. The problem becomes known, is delineated, and stated in terms of either the decision-maker's or the client's goals.
2. Analyze and evaluate the problem. What does the problem mean to the decision-maker and what does it mean to her client? At this point a decision is made as to whether or not a decision should be made.
3. Establish criteria or standards by which a solution will be evaluated or judged as acceptable and adequate to the need. Criteria for evaluation are crucial, and at this stage the value system and aspirations of the individuals involved are built into the process. A decision on criteria and standards must be made prior to the major decision, indicating the sequential nature of the decision-making process.
4. Collect data, more than are necessary. These should be relevant and reproducible.
5. Formulate and select the preferred solution or solutions. Test them in advance. All that has gone on before culminates in a decision—i.e., formulating several solutions, weighing the consequences of each, and selecting a single solution as the one most likely to succeed. The consequences of each solution are weighed and the success of each is predicted by the decision-maker, based on his or her knowledge of the probability of the success of the solutions.
6. The preferred solution is put into effect. This involves

not only implementing but modifying the decision as it becomes operational. Subdecisions have been made in each of the preceding steps, and this step is the sequential outcome of other decisions made during the process.[14]

When a problem is recognized, defined, and solved, the perception as well as the value-system of the decision-maker should be considered. Values give significance and meaning to the problem and determine the degree and nature of the action to be taken.[14] The ability to perceive problems also is related to knowledge of that area in which the problem is located. The decision-making process includes that by which a person implements or makes a decision work. It is recognized as a continuing dynamic process rather than as an occasional event. All judgments that affect a course of action are decisions. The value of a decision stems from the degree to which goals are achieved.

The crucial stage in the decision-making process is the evaluation of proposed solutions to the problem, because it is at this point that the value system and aspirations of the decision-maker have an impact upon the process. The selection of a solution is only part of the process that resulted after several solutions or decisions were formulated, the consequences weighed or probabilities assigned to each, and the solution most likely to be successful was selected. The evaluation stems from the purpose for which the solution was proposed or the reason why the decision was made. During the implementation phase of the decision process, numerous minor decisions may have to be made to modify the solution, as dictated by continuous feedback as the solution becomes operational.[14]

To enhance the caliber of the decisions made, policies may be established that set limitations on the manner and content of decision making. These limitations include the purpose of the system or subsystem, the criterion of rationality of action of members or parts of a system, relevant information, lines of communication, role designations, and time limits.[14] Decision making is a sequential process. Each decision is based upon previous ones. As new information is introduced, the direction of the sequence will change. A decision has an impact on action, in that a course of action may be altered, reversed, discontinued, or continued.[14]

Theoretic formulations from game theory support decision theory and add a dimension to the understanding of the decision process. The theory of games is based upon a sequence of moves or strategies, made by different players, according to a prescribed order, which may depend on the choices made and their outcomes. There exists either a strategy or the probability of a number of strategies for each player. The advantage of communication and cooperation in some games in which players may achieve a pay-off is obvious. The strategies chosen, then, are those most likely to be of maximum benefit to the players. If the nurse and client are viewed as players in a game geared to meet the goals of each, communication and cooperation between nurse and client may facilitate the selection of those strategies or means by which both can achieve their goals or pay-off.[15]

A decision or choice is based on the examination of strategies and the range of possible outcomes. The decision-maker is a complex, living, behaving, goal-seeking system. The living, behaving, adaptive systems of nurse and client are open, both internally and externally, and are negentropic. The interchanges and interactions between systems may cause changes in the nature of each system or subsystem. These changes may have significant implications for the whole system.[16] Internal and external exchanges are transferred by the flow of information (via chemical, cortical, social, or cultural encoding and decoding). Feedback-control facilitates self-regulation and self-direction. Thus the system may change its structure to insure its survival or viability.

PERCEPTION THEORY

In a thriving, living, behaving system in which matter, energy, and information are exchanged within the system as well as with its environment, perception plays an important role. Theories shed light on the origin of the process of perception and provide a rationale for perceptive awareness of the interaction between internal and external environments of the living behaving system or person. The decisions a person makes and his awareness of the choices available to him in a given situation are influenced by his perception of himself as he goes about creating an environment for himself through which he achieves satisfaction and fulfills certain goals. Each person deals with situations according to his own unique system of behavior. It follows that different persons may view a given situation differently and each person will assume that which he perceives is real.

In considering perception, the relationship of the nervous system and the extent to which some aspects of perception do not depend on learning and experience are significant. Day states that perception can be studied in terms of three sets of variables: those in the physical environment, physiologic processes and interactions, and behavioral events. Aspects of perception which serve to mediate overt behavioral responses are the combined function of neural storage, peripheral activity, and central neural events. Central neural storage is a term used to designate the repository of an individual's past as well as current stimulation, with attendant responses resulting in neural events and changes. The overt response of an individual gives rise to kinesthetic, muscular, and mechanical stimulation. The total stimulus complex constitutes a feedback system from response to stimulus input.[17]

Contact between man and environment is accomplished by energy sensitive receptors specifically responsive to certain forms of energy. The characteristics of the stimulation must be transformed into a code for transmission to higher levels of the central nervous system before contact can be established and appropriate adaptive responses initiated. This reception, followed by transformation and energy coding, is the first stage of the perceptual process.[17]

Three classes of receptor cells have been proposed: exteroceptors, interoceptors, and proprioceptors. Exteroceptors are those sensory organ cells that receive energy from the external environment. Interoceptors are cells that respond to changes in pressure, temperature, and pain, including changes in bodily organs and systems within the organism. Proprioceptors are sensitive to energy changes caused by activities involving movement and posture. These three classes of receptor cells selectively pick up stimuli consisting of the total energy changes that occur in the environment, within the organism itself, or are induced by the activities of the organism.[17] Only restricted ranges of environmental energy are necessary to activate the receptors. Also, energy must vary either over time or space; if the stimulus does not change, receptors adapt and become insensitive to it. (Recall the reactions of clients to sensory deprivation and overload during care in highly technical areas of health care facilities.) The sensory system converts the energy of the stimulus and encodes its various properties.[17]

Day has designed a framework to define perception in a coherent manner. His framework draws on: (a) gestalt psychology, which stresses the relationship among stimuli, central neural activity, and state of awareness; (b) stimulation theory, which has drawn attention to variables of a higher order in the array of stimuli; (c) the role of learning in the discrimination of these properties, as prepared by the functionalists who emphasize the part played by learning and perceptual stability in a continually changing environment; and (d) other theories denoting a functional relationship between stimulus-response without considering the underlying process.[17]

The framework developed by Day is as follows: perception is considered in terms of variables in the physical environment, physiologic processes and interactions, and behavior events. Stimulus variables are those that occurred in the person's past as well as current stimulation. Past stimulation, with its attendant responses, results in neural events and changes that can be termed *central neural storage*. A currently acting stimulus induces processes in both the peripheral nervous system (receptors and their structures), called *peripheral neural activity*, and in the central regions (including the cerebral cortex), called *central neural activity*. Central neural storage, peripheral neural activity, and central neural events can be thought of as combining to produce the phenomenal events of perception. These events serve to mediate the overt behavioral response, which gives rise to kinesthetic and muscular stimulation. Mechanical stimulation from the individual's activity is included as part of the total stimulus complex. This constitutes a feedback system from the response to stimulus input.[17] Numerous theories have contributed to an understanding of these perceptual components or events.

Perception may be determined in large part by the learned meanings given to stimuli. Meanings may be inherent in a certain property of stimulation or they may be given by labeling, or by an expectancy induced in the observer. Meanings that are learned affect perception the most when the conditions under which stimulation occurs are ambiguous.[17] Simple percepts lead to more complex perceptual processes associated with the identification of objects, which, in turn, lead to organized perception formed by learning, manipulating, and memorizing previous events.[18]

A perceptive person builds up strong probabilities concerning many expected features of the environment. These greatly affect the particular environmental cues he selects at any one moment for perception and judgment. By checking the accuracy of his percepts through his actions (feedback), he is able to select those cues most likely to give correct or truthful information about the nature of objects and environment. Spatial relationships, locations, colors, distance, movement, would serve as examples.[18] Usually an abundance of information is available and contributes to minimizing error. The process of perception is integrated with processes of identification, classification, and coding. These processes depend upon learning, memory, attention, reasoning, and language. Simple perceptual processes provide data for the operation of more complex processes.[18] Accuracy may be lost when the data are systematized and identified because certain features are ignored, distorted, or over- or under-emphasized. The person must learn to employ the data obtained by perception in such a way that it effectively improves his ability to discriminate. These data may be organized and integrated into complex perceptual systems. The ability to perceive form, position, and the movement of objects in relation to the position and movement of the body is enormously important in understanding adjustments to normal surroundings.[18] To maintain normal perception and cognition, one must be able to perceive change and variation as they occur. The results of research point to profound changes that may result from exposure to homogeneous and unvarying stimulation over a long period of time. The effects of sensory deprivation on the client are apparent to the nurse. This holds true, in a dramatic way, for the client who is unconscious or isolated for some reason. Perception tends to become increasingly less accurate during long periods of observing or responding to a monotonous, repeated stimulation. Many have experienced this impact after they have driven for long, uninterrupted periods on high-speed roadways. There is a physiologic basis for the decrease in alertness and attention due to unvarying stimulation. The discovery of the reticular formation of the brain stem and thalamus, with its variable function, under different types of stimulation, and the control it exercises on cortical functions related to perception, supports the probability that direct attention to various aspects of the environment is related to reticular formation function. This, in turn, may be affected by motivational processes.[18]

Perhaps other cognitive functions may be involved in these complex perceptual processes. It has been shown that information is rarely derived simply from instantaneous perceptions that fade immediately from memory. Impressions are prolonged, at least for a short time, in the primary memory image. This provides continuity in our perceptions of the environment and enhances the use of remembered past experiences as well as the application of reasoning and judgment in evaluating events before reacting or deciding how to act or react. Coding single stimuli and classifying isolated events into perceptual designs provide the basis for understanding the nature of the environment. Life experiences are seldom a function of isolated events but are determined by the continuity of knowledge and experience associated with such perceptions. The inferences a person makes about the nature of objects and events involves knowledge and experiences.[18]

In many life situations, immediate perception may be incorporated in and supplemented by deliberation, judgment, and decision. Individual differences are apparent in many types of perception. People may perceive and react effectively to stimulation without being clearly aware of their total operative percepts. The various reactions demonstrated by different individuals in response to the same situation—witnesses to an accident—supports this statement. Inferences and judgments related to percepts of these witnesses would be as varied as the number of individuals. Motivation and emotion have an effect on arousing, directing, facilitating, or inhibiting the perception of relevant situations and events. But differences in knowledge and acquired skill, of intelligence and ability, are of greater importance than motivational influences in directing attention and promoting efficient discrimination.[18] Accurate perception of the environment is essential to preserve life. While perception may be partially selective, to perform its essential functions efficiently, the selection cannot vary with individual disposition more than to a minor extent.[18]

Vernon also points out that prolonged deprivation of sensory stimulation, and, perhaps even more, of perceptual stimulation, may have far-reaching effects on the normal functioning of cognitive processes. These effects are more severe in some persons than in others. She further states that not only is perception likely to be most rapid and accurate in relevant situations, but expectations are established in such a manner that attention is quickly aroused and directed effectively toward these situations as soon as they occur. While there is a tendency to respond to novel and unexpected events, more deliberate perception and inference may be necessary to gain a full understanding of the situation before action takes place. A fundamental tendency is the ability to respond to a constantly varying environment. Movement is considered a frequent environmental variation. It is supposed that there is an innate tendency to perceive the movements of people. It is possible that learning through experiences may influence the inception of these perceptions—as in the perception of smiling faces. These perceptions can be enormously refined and improved through learning.[18]

Vernon concludes that perception begins with the responses of cell units in the sensory mechanism to stimuli.

These responses are then integrated into patterns and con-figurations that are fundamentally significant in perception. She hypothesizes that the infant possesses an innate tendency to perceive form as well as the natural environment in terms of objects and that this tendency begins to operate as his experiences with objects develop. The infant has a natural tendency to perceive a spatial continuum within which objects are spatially related to himself and to each other. It is supposed that from infancy upwards, the child builds up complex integrations (also called schemata) by means of which what is perceived at any moment is related to memories and knowledge, particularly those obtained through the active ex-perience of manipulating objects and moving through the en-vironment.[18] The process of reasoning and of conceptual classification comes to bear on these integrations.

Perception of objects, particularly in the complex en-vironmental settings with which we are normally concerned, develops comparatively slowly. This development depends on the capacity to sort out essential aspects from a multitude of irrelevant detail. The nature and identity of new and unfa-miliar objects are explored and discovered by the child him-self by applying not only his habitual activities but also vari-ations of these to find out what can be done with the objects. Carefully, he watches to see what happens to an object when he lets it fall to the floor. He forms a notion of what action to perform and what its outcome may be. Integration or schemata of perception are involved, covering categories of objects (appearance, behavior, use) associated together as they relate to each other in complex organizations. Imme-diate perception is integrated with respect to conceptual rea-soning.[18] The capacity to extract such general qualities as size, number, volume, weight, height, and to judge these, irrespective of the objects and settings in which they occur, requires reasoning. This is an essential component of judg-ment and involves the realization that these attributes may remain constant in spite of changes in appearance or setting. Vernon gives a useful example of this idea when she notes that the volume of water remains constant when it is poured from a wide container into a narrow one, even though the level of water in the latter is higher. A child may observe the obvious height of the water level. His judgment of the volume of water in the container is overweighted by his perception of the water level, and he may note that the volume of water is different. There are other situations in which immediate perception is uncorrected by reasoning.[18]

Vernon continues her discussion of perception through experiences by stating that the ability to modify immediate perception through reasoning is generally supposed to develop as a person matures, although at the stage at which it begins to develop, experience and learning may affect it considerably. While the capacity to identify and recognize is determined by maturation to a considerable extent, experience is known to play an important role, providing information about the nature and characteristics of objects.[18] The identification of these objects—general qualities and type—is based upon information.

The following suppositions relate to perception through experience:

1. Generalization of learning from one situation to another could occur in so far as situations or events become organized within the same schemata in such a manner that present percepts are filled out and extended by memories of relevant past experiences and appropriate responses are made available.
2. The utilization of class categories is a significant feature of improved identification from the second year of life. Children and adults learn to distinguish the invariant qualities of a class of events or objects (on which identification is based) from chance variations resulting from changes in the background situation.
3. Verbal discrimination plays a significant part in the process of naming, labeling, and coding. Verbal information furthers the control of immediate perception by reasoning processes.[18]

It does not necessarily follow, even if one perceives with a reasonable degree of accuracy or truthfulness, that shapes and contours are exact replicas of the stimulus pattern falling on the eye. The forms of which persons are actually aware may be reconstructions from sensory data. There are many aspects of complex situations provided by the natural environment of which persons are not accurately aware. The stimulus pattern gives rise to cues from which the appearance of objects and their spatial setting can be inferred. Perceptions of form in everyday life may not involve accurate discrimination of minute detail, though the capacity to do this is available. This capacity may be utilized in selected scientific activities or in precision measurements. Generally there is an over-abundance of sensory information, much of which is corroborative. The observer must select what is relevant to his identification of the objects and events he visualizes and initiate appropriate reaction. The perceiver utilizes schematized knowledge as to the type of situation and the relevant response pattern. There may be occasions in which information is restricted or conflicting. It may be so abundant that one must sift for relevancy and discard that which is irrelevant. In situations such as this, the perceiver makes inferences about the real nature of the situation or about the objects presented to him.[18] The nurse experiences this when she must gather data on an unconscious person and no one is available to give information about his predicament. Other examples are data available about an infant if there is no adult with him to interpret, or if a person—either the nurse or the client—speaks a foreign language, a highly technical language, or if the language is distorted. By making inferences the observer goes beyond immediate sensory data and extracts information that gives the truest impression of the nature of the situation in which immediately perceptible aspects of the stimulus occur. Inference may override erroneous impressions given by visual illustrations.[18] There are conditions, however, in which inferences related to the identity of objects and events are erroneous; for example: those seen in dim light, from great distances, or for short periods of time. In terms of the perception of words, understanding their meaning seems to be more important than their frequency.[18]

The relationship between attention and perception has been studied by some investigators who have demonstrated that there may be a process of attending that operates independently of perceptual processes. Previously, it was thought that if a person attended a stimulus, he automatically perceived it. Physiologic and psychologic investigations have identified a special center in the brain which is concerned with attention. A decline in attention and in interference with normal perception has been noted in persons partially or completely deprived of variable sensory stimulation.[18]

While observers are prone to make inferences from fragments of information and these inferences are influenced by what the observer expects to perceive, focusing attention on particular events or aspects of the stimulus, and the expectation that certain types of stimulation may occur, may identify stimuli which, under other circumstances, would be ignored completely.[18]

The implications for the nurse are many. Continual striving to increase the observational field, as well as to increase her knowledge about human behavior and the human situation, could enhance her ability to collect data and increase the accuracy of her inferences concerning the client. Thus, she can make educated estimates about gaps in data and pursue specific information to fill them. The process used to select data, reactions to data or stimuli, and her focus on particular events related to the availability or absence of data is a decision process.

While the foregoing discussion has centered more on perception as it relates to form, objects, languages, space, and movement, an important perceptual schema that differs considerably is the perception of people, their emotions, and their actions. Vernon believes that from the earliest years people perceived other people, their faces, and their behavior in a manner unique to these types of percepts. A special schemata has evolved within which these percepts are integrated. The unique aspect of these percepts is that the perceivers are mainly aware of the intentions, emotions, and personality characteristics of persons; only to a minor extent are they aware of the details of the physical characteristics (appearance and behavior) of these people. Stimulus patterns involved in the perception of persons are more complex and extensive than those on which the perception of objects is based. From early infancy, previous knowledge and expectations concerning the actions and motives of people are highly significant, and from their perceptions of physical properties, children learn to make inferences about significant characteristics of people and their behavior.[18] As they develop their perception of persons, infants and children look predominantly into the eyes and upper part of a person's face. Relative to the perception of emotion, facial expressions related to somewhat temporary emotions are differentiated from perceptions of more lasting characteristics by which familiar people are identified and impressions of their personality characteristics are based. Emotions frequently felt and expressed may give rise to permanent facial characteristics, such as wrinkles around the eyes and in the forehead.[18]

As to the accuracy with which emotional expressions are perceived, studies indicate that emotions judged from facial expressions are easier to differentiate if they correspond to the extremes of pleasant/unpleasant or attention/rejection. This does not mean that this is the extent to which perceptions of emotional expressions are accurate in every day situations. Facial expression is a dynamic and constantly changing characteristic. It is accompanied by action, expressive gestures, and changes in vocal intonation. Studies have shown that infants understand the emotions of others, i.e., fear, anger. Of course, this depends on whether the relationship between the emotion that is felt and its outward expression is consistent.[18]

Perceptual data on which assessments of emotions other than one's own are based are extremely complex. It is difficult, if not impossible, to isolate any one facial feature that is consistently associated with a particular emotional expression. Some expressions can be identified readily, such as a smile or frown. There seems to be little basis for some prevailing associations—a high forehead indicates high intelligence, for example. Again, the implication is obvious, in that

far-reaching judgments or inferences, based on little or selected data, may be totally inaccurate. Prejudices and stereotypes have resulted from this tendency to select certain facial
characteristics and bodily poses. Some associations between
facial and personality characteristics may result in social
stereotypes. It is generally considered, for example, that a
smiling face with an upcurved mouth indicates a good-
tempered person. These stereotyped associations vary in different societies and in different groups within these societies.
Often, stereotypes are more likely to be attributed to strangers or foreigners. The more resemblance there is between a
stranger and a familiar person the more likely the stereotype
will be favorable.[18]

Floyd Allport[19] contributed some insights to the understanding of the nature of perception when he analyzed it
from a systems viewpoint. He compares organisms and machines (cybernetics) and notes that each has a common feature—input and output. For the organism, input is the stimulus (energy, food, water), while output is the work done by
the effector or mechanism. The system's internal operation is
akin to metabolism—that point of operation connecting input
and output. Psychologically speaking, input would refer to
the energy derived from stimulated receptors while output is
the coordination of the action of effectors called *behaviors*.
Both machines and organisms use working energy, power,
and raw materials as input and convert this to service and
finished product as outputs. There are special energetic units
that usually operate through some subsystem referred to as
information. This information can be compared to the stim-
ulations received by the organism through its receptors, since
it affects the action of the machine or organism in a controlled manner. Random stimuli or energetic events that do
not become effective toward output bombard the organism,
and are referred to as *noise*. Information which affects output is considered negative entropy or organization; random
disturbances of noise are entropy. The designer of a machine
strives to keep noise to a minimum while the organism (particularly the human organism) strives to reduce the propor-
tion of random, uncoordinated, or disorganized behavior

through perception, reasoning, or learning.[19]

Human beings communicate with and control one another, within the organization of society, by spoken word, using mechanical transmitting devices, such as the telephone or telegraph. Information can be communicated to a machine to fulfill a task. The communicator of information to parts or subsystems of a mechanical system enables the parts to be synchronized to the demands of the task—rate of output is controlled by the system to contribute to purposeful goals. The feedback mechanism enhances the interdependence of parts of the system, keeping it in a steady state as the flow from input goes through it. Its function is to regulate and control the operation of the entire system. The amount of information fed back to the main part of the system is always the extent to which there remains a gap between the actual and desired condition. It corrects many fluctuations in the operation of a complicated mechanism, with a minimal amount of inefficiency or loss. The feedback principle is prevalent in natural, socially evolved, and deliberately constructed systems.[19]

The living organism has an input and an output. It has receptors into which information is fed. There are effectors in the organism—muscles, glands, etc., as well as an arrangement for integrating, storing, and transferring information between input and output. Storage and recollection are located in the physiologic mechanism through which information is retained, recognized, and recalled. Messages are not only transmitted from the outside but from within the system through established pathways. These messages are delivered by the kinesthetic receptors and proprioceptors of the organism. The nervous system, like the computer, operates on relatively small amounts of energy in which the structural character of the operations is circular rather than a straight line.[19] But, the operator designates the purpose and is the basis for the feedback subsystem. The purpose is not in any part of the system, but is the end for which the system was designed.

If living behaving systems are viewed as aggregates of designated ongoing events, they will be found to have a self-limited, self-closed, and circular character. These same forms of events apply to systems at a higher level—to all collective or societal aggregates in which organisms operate, including economic, political, and other systems in which men or machines play a part. Circular operating structures may be conceived as interrelated by the same set of principles that enter into their individual construction and operation.[19] Thus, systems theory, particularly theories related to machine and communication systems, shed some light on the study of the nature and process of perception. These theories have enhanced the knowledge of how the brain and nervous system operate.

To understand meaning in perception, it must be approached through the perceived character of objects and situations that have meaning to us. There are other phases of meaning, but that which gives us the unique characteristics of objects and situations is the one most central to the entire perceptual process. Meaning has a wider scope than the perceived character of objects. It enters into processes in addition to that of perception. Meaning is the very appropriateness with which perceiving, remembering, and acting are explained. When we perceive, remember, think, or will, we assign meaning.[19] Thus, perception plays a crucial role in life, in general, for it is the sole means through which we can gather information about the world around us. It is also the only means by which nurse and client gather data about each other. In turn, these data are assigned designated values and then used to fulfill the purposes of nursing.

SUMMARY

General systems theory has developed through the special attention it received in various areas of science and has contributed to the general framework within which natural phenomena are explained. System is seen as any recognizable delimited aggregate of interconnected dynamic elements that are in some way interdependent and continue to operate together according to certain laws to produce a characteristic total effect. It is concerned with activity and preserves a kind of integration and unity. A particular system can be recognized as distinct from others to which it may be dynamically related. Systems may be complex in that they may be composed of interdependent subsystems, each of which, though less autonomous than the entire aggregate, is fairly distinguishable in its operation.[18]

Systems are of two types—open and closed. A closed system is one in which no energy is received from an outside source and which does not provide energy to its surroundings. Open systems are those whose actions provide a continuous product output. The nature of the system is such that after any disturbance in input, its constant and time-independent characteristics may be restored, maintained, and/or reestablished. Although never in true equilibrium, the system maintains itself in a steady state, that is, neither static nor motionless. Instead it is marked by ceaseless activity and a change in the specific materials involved. The organism maintains its steady state by the fact that degradative processes in the cells are being continually compensated for by synthetic and anabolic processes. This work requires energy, and, therefore, the organism requires nourishment merely to exist—to maintain itself in a steady state quite apart from the energy that goes into effective work upon the environment. Open systems have the characteristic of equifinality, which is the ability to attain steady states independent of initial conditions. The growth or maturation of a living behaving system is an example.[19] Although the entropic process never becomes reversed and continues to some extent in all systems, in open systems a remarkable state of affairs occurs; for the time being and in certain parts or aspects of the system, entropy ceases (a measure of disorder). The measure or degree to which the system or part of the system stays away from entropy is called *negative entropy* (a measure of order).[19] Communication within the system is handled by a feedback mechanism that enhances its viability and its purposefulness. Decisions are an important component because of the selection choices and alternatives needed to maintain a steady state. If the system is a living behaving system, as it is in the case of a nurse and her client, communication within parts of and between the system and its environment is accomplished through perception. Perception, too, can be understood from a system point of view—at least in part—because input or messages are encoded, processed, and decoded with feedback adjustments so that awareness and adaptation to the environment are accomplished.

Thus, the nurse, as a unique perceiving person in interaction with a client who is also a unique perceiving person, comprises that system of nursing whose goal is to meet the health care and nursing needs of citizens. Perceptions of both the nurse and client are fashioned from life experiences and knowledge, and each must be available (at least in part) to the other and communicated so that problems and needs related to health and its maintenance can be identified. The more information available, the greater the knowledge of alternatives, the keener the ability to predict outcome, the more effective the selection from alternatives, and the more successful the solution. The amount, quality, and focus of the nurse's knowledge and experience has an impact on the quality of her perception in a nursing situation. Similarly, the client's knowledge, experiences, and life style have an impact on how he thinks of his health, his predicament, and of the nurse as a helping person. The nursing process is designed to meet the client's need for health and nursing care. It is a data-gathering, decision process with a built-in feedback mechanism in the form of evaluation and modification. Thus, the nurse has the means with which to collect, designate meaning to, and make inferences about information, verify these inferences, plan to remedy designated problems or deficits, select the most appropriate alternative, and then implement this plan. Evaluation of the outcome, with modification, maintains the interaction in a viable state, and focuses efforts in the direction of a solution. This may result in reassessment, replacement, a change in implementation, then reevaluation. The nursing process is cyclic. Using it in nursing practice is strategic to enhance the relevance and purpose of the nurse-client interaction.

In summary, the cyclic and parallel nature of the following theories as well as the nursing process itself are illustrated in the diagrammatic sketch:

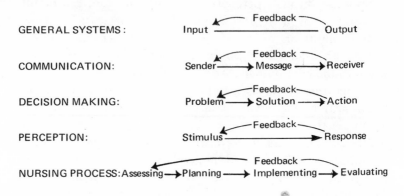

GENERAL SYSTEMS: Input ——— Feedback ——— Output

COMMUNICATION: Sender —→ Message —→ Receiver (Feedback)

DECISION MAKING: Problem —→ Solution —→ Action (Feedback)

PERCEPTION: Stimulus —→ Response (Feedback)

NURSING PROCESS: Assessing —→ Planning —→ Implementing —→ Evaluating (Feedback)

REFERENCES

1. Banathy B H: Instructional Systems. Palo Alto, Calif, Fearon Publishers, 1968, pp 1-14
2. von Bertalanffy L: General System Theory. New York, George Braziller Co, 1968, pp 37-38, 142-143
3. System Change, and Conflict. Edited by N J Demerath, R Peterson. New York, The Free Press, 1967, p 122
4. Hazzard M: An overview of systems theory. Nurs Clin N Am 26:383-462, 1971
5. Simon H: The Sciences of the Artificial. Cambridge, M I T Press, 1969, p 52, 55, 77, 95-97, 112
6. Raymond R: Communication, entropy, and life. Modern Systems Research for the Behavioral Scientist. Edited by W. Buckley. Chicago, Aldine Publishing Co, 1968, p 160
7. Mackay D: The informational analysis of questions and commands.[6] pp 204-208, 206
8. Buckley, W: Information, Communication, and Meaning,[6] p 119
9. De Fleur M: Theories of Mass Communication. New York, David McKay Co, Inc, 1966, pp 91-94
10. Rapaport A: The promise and pitfalls of information theory.[6] pp 137-142
11. Schrödinger E: Order, disorder, and entropy.[6] pp 144-145
12. Frick F C: The application of information theory in behavioral studies.[6] pp 182-183
13. Ackoff R: Towards a behavioral theory of communication, Modern System Research for the Behavioral Scientist. Edited by W Buckley. Chicago, Aldine Publishing Co, 1968, pp 209-218
14. Griffiths D: Administration as decision-making, Chap 6, In Administrative Theory in Education. Edited by A Halpin. London, The Macmillan Co, 1958, pp 123-140
15. Rapaport A: Critiques of game theory.[6] pp 474-489

16. Buckley W: Society as a Complex Adaptive System.[6] pp 490-513

17. Day R H: Perception. Dubuque, Iowa, Wm C Brown Company, 1966, pp 6-9, 34, 42-43

18. Vernon M: Perception through Experience. London, England, Methuen and Co, Ltd, 1970, pp 1-240

19. Allport F: Theories of Perception and the Concept of Structure. New York, John Wiley and Sons, 1955, pp 477-478, 485, 493, 526, 566

chapter three

Analysis of
the Components of
the Nursing Process

Based upon its theoretic framework, each component or phase of the nursing process will be developed and analyzed, according to the persons, both nurses and clients, involved in the process. The goal of analysis will be to suggest the components of the process appropriate to nursing actions, considering such factors as cultural background, age, level of wellness, degree of illness, as well as socioeconomic and educational levels. The unique aspect of each component as well as their interrelationships will be considered. The components of the nursing process follow a logical progression, but two or more may be operational at the same time. The time span for using the process will vary with the client's situation and may portray immediate and long-term goals.

The nurse and client are viewed as partners in nursing, a subsystem of the health care system. Each person is viewed as a unique member of the family and the community—units of a social system. The nurse draws heavily on perception, communication, and decision-making in her use of the nursing process. The client utilizes these skills in his role by participating in assessing, planning, implementing, and evaluating his care.

The four phases or components of the nursing process used in this text are useful and inclusive. They incorporate many ideas of other authors who designate other, though similar, steps in the nursing process, the four components of which—assessing, planning, implementing, and evaluating—are the core of effective nurse actions. The nursing process is very vital and on-going, enhancing the level of success in solving client health and nursing care problems, utilizing the nurse's knowledge and skill to identify and solve client care problems, and solving them quickly, accurately, and economically. This implies a minimum waste of nursing personnel effort and facilities. The client gets the best care directly, in the shortest time possible from the person who is best able to identify and solve his problem or problems.

The nursing process is systematized, appropriate for the well person or family or for the acutely or chronically ill. It can be used by nurse practitioners in whatever setting the client or family is in. It is important for the nurse to designate client problems, but it is just as important that she refrain from creating problems where none exist. Utilizing a logical, goal-directed process safeguards against creating problems. There is a cyclic nature to the nursing process, and the movement is constant between and among its components (Fig.1).

The skills the nurse must have to use the nursing process are: intellectual, interpersonal, and technical. Intellectual skills entail problem-solving, critical thinking, and making nursing judgments. Interpersonal skills are related to the ability to communicate, listen, and convey interest, compassion, knowledge, and information, and to obtain needed data in a manner that enhances the individuality of the client as a person. These skills foster relationships with the client, his family, co-workers, and colleagues. Technical skills relate to methods, procedures, and the machines used to bring about specific results or the desired behavioral responses of the client. Decisions and decision-making are a part of every component.

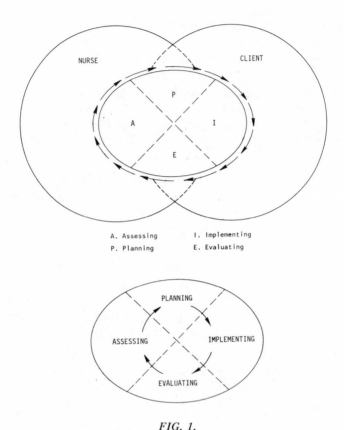

A. Assessing   I. Implementing

P. Planning   E. Evaluating

FIG. 1.

Involvement in the nursing process assumes concern for persons, problems, places, and health. To engage successfully in this process, the following premises are pertinent.

1. A person is a human being endowed with worth and dignity.
2. A person has basic human needs that must be met.
3. Problems result when needs are partially met or unmet—due to limitations in physical, emotional, spiritual, social, and economic capability and the availability of resources.

4. Inability to fulfill one's basic human needs may entail the intervention of another individual who can help a person meet his needs or fill the need directly until such time as the person can resume that responsibility for himself.

5. A person or family presenting themselves for health care desires a client-centered approach that enhances their value and seeks solutions to their health and nursing care problems in the most effective, yet economic manner.

6. The nurse is interested in rendering high quality service to persons and families, no matter what their life style, economic status, or cultural or religious beliefs might be.

7. To utilize the nursing process and develop goal-directed nursing care plans the nurse must have up-to-date knowledge of theories from the physical, biologic, social, and behavioral sciences and must have mastered a knowledge of nursing as well.

8. The practice of nursing involves the ability to focus on another person and requires the full attention and energy of the nurse when she is engaged in the practice of nursing.

9. The heart of the nurse-client interaction is the development of a helping relationship in which the nurse fosters the client's personal development and growth through empathetic understanding, faith in the client's growth potential, respecting and caring for and about the client in an unconditional manner, willingly being available, and freely being one's genuine self.[1]

10. Successful nursing practice results from continued study—both formal and informal—and from an ongoing evaluation of one's self-development and nursing practice, with plans to maximize strengths and minimize limitations.

11. The person or family demonstrate a willingness to share information, feelings, and concerns so that problems can be identified and solutions sought.

12. The nurse strives to meet her own self-development through the practice of nursing.

13. Every citizen has the right to quality health and nursing

care rendered with interest, competence, and compassion.

14. Nurse practitioners need to focus on preventing disease,
maintaining wellness, and rendering care to the sick.

ASSESSING

The assessment phase begins with the nursing history and
ends with a nursing diagnosis. The purpose of this phase is to
identify and obtain data about the client that will enable the
nurse and/or the client or his family to designate problems
relating to wellness and illness. If problems exist, then the
first step toward a solution is to identify them.

The nurse's function is to assess wellness or illness and
their extent. In some instances, this ability may mean the
difference between life or death for the client. In contrast to
goals of other members of the health profession, the nurse
does involve herself with basic human needs that affect
the *total* person rather than one aspect, one problem, or
a limited segment of need fulfillment. The objective is to
meet all basic human needs. The nurse will try to satisfy
the needs of each person individually. Her effectiveness in
assessing these needs depends upon her knowledge of
basic human needs, a solid base of anatomy and physiology, a
knowledge of human behavior, major causes of morbidity
and mortality, human growth and development, personality
development, and knowledge of basic pathophysiology and
psychopathology. A knowledge of various cultures with their
beliefs and patterns, a knowledge of major religions of the
world and the obligations and patterns of the faithful following these religions, a knowledge of family and social organization and the economic patterns for that segment of society
in which the nurse practices, as well as variations in other
segments—state, regional, national, and international—are
needed.

The nurse must first determine which needs are to be
assessed, what and how much information will be needed,
and from whom and where she can obtain this information or
data.

Nursing care rendered in conjunction with the client or clients is directed toward maintaining a state of wellness, care of the sick, or both. Where wellness cannot be realized, supportive care is given so that the client can function to maximum capability.

It must be remembered that a need is not a problem in itself. The word *need* is used in many ways, sometimes as a noun and sometimes as a verb. It is used to denote a lack of something or to mean a requisite for bodily or psychic functioning. It is used frequently in everyday conversation. A need is not necessarily a problem, but a client can develop a problem when a basic human need is not met, or filled only partially. The terms *nursing need* and *nursing problem,* as heard in conversations and as they appear in the literature, refer to a nursing order, the action or intervention by a nurse to solve or resolve an assessed client problem. The word *need* denotes necessity or use for. The terms used in this text are *basic human need* and *client problem.*

The nurse may use a variety of theoretic models to designate basic human needs. Maslow's[2] Hierarchy of Needs and Erikson's[3] Eight Ages of Man both are popular and useful models. The discussion of assessment will focus on these models. While categories of needs are general in nature, the nurse must assess individual or particular aspects of each.

Basic human needs refer to those all people must satisfy to enhance their images of themselves as persons. The first category of needs, as distinguished by Maslow, are physiologic—food, oxygen, physical activity, rest, elimination, water, and sexual satisfaction. All are present at birth except the need for sexual satisfaction, which differs because it is active only intermittently and can be satisfied by substitute measures.

The second category comprises safety and security, such as requirements for sameness, sureness, familiarity, and trustworthiness in people, things, places, and events. The third category is the need for love or belonging, including affection, warmth, kindness, and consideration in human relationships. The fourth is the need for self-esteem, such as respect, status, prestige, and a good reputation. For the child, these needs are met by significant others through their approval and confidence in the child, their respect of him, and the fact they regard him as a valuable person. The adult derives satisfaction from successful accomplishments in work and other activity. A sense of accomplishment carries with it feelings of adequacy, competency, and mastery. Needs for love and esteem form stepping stones to self-actualization, the fifth category. It is also viewed as the state of becoming, and involves the ability to control oneself, one's destiny, and one's needs rather than being controlled by them.

A person never outgrows his physiologic needs or his need for security, love, and esteem. Persons are motivated by all of these needs, but more so by some than by others at any given time. At times of stress, crisis, or illness, problems may arise in meeting some or all of these needs.[4] Illness does not mean these needs do not have to be satisfied; in fact, it may create heavier demands for fulfilling particular needs, the way in which they are met, or even by whom they would be met and when.

Physiologic needs must be met in preference to others only when the deprivation is life threatening. As soon as the threat diminishes, attention must be paid to other categories of needs. Factors that influence needs include age and sex; intellectual, emotional, educational, social, and financial capability; level of wellness or illness; type, location, and extent of pathophysiology and/or psychopathology; and the type, availability, and the effectiveness of the therapeutic regimen.

It is not possible to separate the physical, psychologic, emotional, spiritual, educational, social, and cultural aspects of a person. This is attempted academically, but in reality, a person is a unified entity. Rarely does a client have a physical problem that does not give rise to a psychologic component, a social and economic impact, nor does a psychologic problem exist without a physical response to situations experienced. Need fulfillment is a motivating force. Needs motivate behavior directed toward achieving satisfaction. In addition to wholeness, each person meets his particular needs in an individual manner, contributing to the unique characteristics of an individual.

By becoming aware of and by gaining knowledge about one's own inner experiences, a person develops a reliable basis from which the inner experiences of others can be assessed. Within everyone, there is a basic drive for growth and development in the direction of optimal realization of his potential. His motivation and his perceptions are a trustworthy basis for action constructive for him. The nurse can facilitate and nourish the client's own basic drive for widening development. Any attempt to force this motivation into being or into activity will usually defeat its own purpose. The client is responsible for himself. The nurse really cannot be responsible for him, although she is accountable and responsible for her own behavior toward him.[1]

To focus on one aspect, such as the physical, to the exclusion of the others, or to ignore the hypothesis that what affects any one aspect of an individual inevitably affects all other aspects, is to assess the client's problem in a limited manner. The limited perspective could create problems rather than diagnose or solve problems for the client.

Deprivations of needs, particularly those relating to food and oxygen, create a state within the person which demands satisfaction to survive. The person will focus his behavior exclusively toward obtaining food or air. In *Man's Search for Meaning* the author, Viktor Frankl,[5] discusses the impact of hunger during imprisonment and tells how prisoners dream of food and their exhaustive attempts to relieve their hunger. The fact that hunger is a total experience, not limited to a physical reaction alone, explains why some persons place a high priority on meeting basic life-sustaining needs. A starving person can hardly be expected to care for intellectual and interpersonal pursuits, economic advancement, and social status. Similar situations have been witnessed and experienced at times of natural disasters, such as floods, explosions, and other environmental upheavals. Once these needs are partially or completely satisfied, however, the person tries to fulfill other categories of his needs. By their reactions and behavior, people demonstrate their needs for safety and security, love or belonging, esteem, and, in the adult, self-fulfillment. The nurse has observed manifestations of low self-esteem, depression, withdrawal, hostile or aggressive behavior, and anxiety.

When considering the total person, it will be noted that he has needs in common with others. While these common needs are acknowledged, each person is still unique, whether he or she is a client or the nurse. The personality of every individual is unique; the combination of qualities and characteristics he possesses, his set of values, ways of reacting, interacting, and transacting can only be attributed to this one person alone. In some ways, his specific needs and reactions may be similar to patterns of other persons, but each has some characteristic entirely different from that of any other person.

Another useful model is the eight stages of development toward maturity proposed by Erikson. Summarized briefly, these are:

1. *Basic Trust versus Basic Mistrust*: developing a sense of trust and security derived from affection and the gratification of needs during infancy—from birth to 1 year of age. Hope is the outcome.
2. *Autonomy versus Shame and Doubt*: achieving a sense of autonomy in which the child views himself as an individual in his own right, beginning from his early childhood years (1 to 4 years old). Will power is the outcome.
3. *Initiative versus Guilt*: developing a sense of initiative, and a period of vigorous testing; imagination of adult behaviors occurs during the ages 4 to 5. A sense of purpose is the outcome.
4. *Industry versus Inferiority*: developing a sense of industry and of duty and accomplishment, understanding real tasks; developing academic and social competence occurs during school age (6 to 11). Competence is the outcome.
5. *Identity versus Role Confusion*: A sense of identity, clarifying who one is and what one's role is, develops during the adolescent years (12 to 15). Fidelity is the outcome to be achieved.
6. *Intimacy versus Isolation*: A sense of intimacy, the ability to establish close personal relationships with members of both sexes begins to develop at the age of 15 years. Love is the lasting outcome.
7. *Generativity versus Stagnation*: Parental sense, produc-

tivity, and creativity for others as well as one's self; a sense of generativity develops during adulthood. Care is the outcome to be achieved.

8. *Ego Integrity versus Despair*: A sense of integrity, acceptance of the dominant ideals of one's culture, a sense of continuity with the past, present, and future, and the meaningfulness of life develops with adulthood and maturity. Wisdom is the outcome.[3]

The developmental stages of man provide a basis for understanding the client and a framework for determining wellness. The person must be viewed as a whole, with consideration given to his uniqueness, and the variation that characterizes his patterns of action, his view of himself, and his view of others. Going one step further, it would be useful to consider the unique characteristics of the client and nurse, rendering their interactions and their relationships also unique. Perhaps, this is what is "unique" about nursing.

Inherent in the idea that each person is unique—demonstrating qualities, characteristics, needs common to other persons, and, at the same time, manifesting a particular difference, is to accept one's own individuality. The nurse must first understand her own strengths, her limitations, her pattern of response, her views, and her values, before she can be receptive to and accept those of her client. Her ability to assess and deal with her own behavior and that of the client presupposes a knowledge of human behavior and her belief in prevalent assumptions about behavior. Brown and Fowler compiled a useful list of these assumptions, which include a knowledge that:

1. A person's total response to a stimulus constitutes his behavior. The responses may generate from sources within or outside the individual—for example, a person who develops a fever in response to invasion by pneumococci or who shivers when he is in a cold room. Further, there is a covert as well as an overt aspect to each behavioral response. Covert responses include a person's thoughts, feelings, and motivations, while behaviors include verbalizations and human actions.

2. A person's behavior is governed by his available energy and is always within range of the maximum energy with which he is endowed. His behavior cannot manifest more energy than that which is available to him, although this quantity varies with his energy potential at any given time. Individuals differ from each other in their energy potential for behavior. Factors that might influence the availability of energy include: caloric intake, metabolic rate, atmospheric conditions—humidity, temperature, barometric pressure, sensory overload, age, sex, concept of self, timing and number of demands upon the person at any given time, and his view of the value of these demands.

3. Behavior has a purpose, even though this purpose is not always obvious. The person may be trying to accomplish something. This accomplishment or lack of it may be in terms of gain, loss, or in maintaining one's self or situation.

4. A person's response to a particular situation is the best of that which he is capable of at a particular time. This does not preclude that the person can respond differently or more effectively by learning other patterns of response. These responses would be applicable to other client situations, particularly if there is some similarity between the situations. Knowing that a person is responding in the best way possible at a given moment makes it easier for the nurse to accept herself as well as the client as a person, whether or not she approves of a particular behavioral response.

5. A person's perception of what is happening to him has a greater influence on his behavior than what is actually happening or how it is interpreted by another person. The nurse must validate inferences about the client with him. The nurse's intentions and goals must be shared with the client and must be verified and accepted if her diagnoses and plans for action are to be successful.

6. Each person has a potential for striving forward. Since motivation to proceed in this direction is inherent within the person, efforts can be directed to stimulate and activate those forces having a positive influence. It may be necessary to designate basic human needs that must be fulfilled, whatever their category, as a precursor to meet-

ing more mature needs. Efforts to stimulate advancement must be based upon an accurate assessment of the current status of the person's needs, which will serve as a baseline in evaluating change and the direction of change.

7. A person satisfies most of his needs in an interpersonal manner with other persons and/or groups of persons, each demonstrating dependent, independent, and interdependent behavior. The quality and quantity of these manifestations change as the person progresses from infancy to adulthood. Their quality increases as each person experiences and copes with human situations as he strives for self-fulfillment or self-actualization.[6]

The nurse, as the helping person, must be willing to understand the client from his own frame of reference. She senses and seeks to understand what is real and meaningful to him at any point in time and must know how he sees things, or feels about himself. She is sensitive to his conscious feelings and the meanings underlying his outward communication. The nurse maintains a clear distinction between meaning that originates in herself and that which originates in her client. She attempts to understand his meaning at a particular moment with the idea that this understanding is subject to correction and change as new data become available.[1] Caring for and about the client is unqualified; that is, no conditions are attached to it. The client does not need to earn approval or liking by expressing some desires and suppressing others, by portraying certain attitudes or beliefs and denying others, or by being one type of person and not another. This rules out the need to label clients as *uncooperative-cooperative, demanding-docile,* etc.[1] These beliefs are conveyed to the client during all phases of the nursing process. Efforts to establish a helping relationship begin with the first nurse-client interaction, at the time the client enters the health care system, and it continues as long as this interaction is needed.

In addition to knowledge of basic human needs, assumptions about human behavior, and characteristics of a helping relationship, the nurse needs a strong knowledge of anatomy and physiology, chemistry, physics, microbiology, psychology, sociology, human growth and development, mathematics, literature, art, philosophy, pathophysiology, psycho-pathology, and theology. The content of these courses provides the basis for her knowledge of man in his world, of the person who is well (including self-development of the nurse), and, in addition, provides a basis for recognizing a change in a person's state of wellness. The selection of specific principles from these biologic, physical, and behavioral sciences provides the rationale for the nurse's actions, facilitates her decision making, and enhances her person-centered interactions. Specifically, basic principles and theories from selected biologic, physical, and behavioral sciences will provide the framework for assessing the client's health status and his need for nursing intervention.

A framework of factors to be assessed will focus on those common to all persons. The nurse must adapt and adjust this framework to incorporate specifics which determine the unique aspects of a particular person and/or family. The collection of data related to these factors will also be devised creatively by the nurse to suit settings in which she is functioning. For example: factors for assessment may have dimensions different for the school nurse, the office nurse, the nurse in the community health center, the nurse in a health maintenance organization, the nurse in a nursing home, the nurse in a rural setting, an urban setting, in an acute care setting or chronic care setting, or the nurse working with persons of a particular age group, such as infants, adolescents, or oldsters, with men or women, or with those who are sightless, deaf, or mentally retarded. Initially the nurse starts with a prescribed list of factors, but she should exercise her intellect and creativity in developing an in-depth list, based on her observations, experiences, and an analysis of factors portrayed by clients with similar problems.

Among these factors are those relating to age, sex, education, growth and development, socioeconomic, cultural and religious elements, biologic and physical status, emotional status, coping patterns, interactional patterns, life style, employment, the client's view of health and illness as it relates to himself and his family.[7-9] In addition, consideration must be given to the client's expectations of health care and his awareness of the roles of health-care practitioners, particularly that of the nurse; the physical, social, emotional, and ecologic environment in which he lives and works; and the human and material resources available and accessible to him.

When assessing factors related to age and sex, the nurse should know the needs, roles, expectations, and behaviors relative to infancy, childhood, adolescence, adulthood, and senesence for male and female persons. Maslow's Hierarchy of Needs,[2] Erikson's Eight Ages of Man,[3] and Duvall's Family Development[10] are a useful guide to the collection of meaningful data and provide a basis for validating inferences and designating problems. Age and sex are extremely important factors when considering a person, whether he or she is the client or nurse. These factors are combined with all others and influence each other significantly.

When assessing factors relating to the needs of persons from different racial groups, the nurse needs to know their customs, rites, rituals, roles, traditions, expectations, and views, particularly those of persons living in the United States.

When assessing religious factors, the nurse must know the various religions of this era as well as the beliefs, rites, and rituals of each. A knowledge of the rules freeing individuals from participating in religious rites and rituals because of illness or handicap with implications, of the rites and rituals of the different religions, as they apply or are available to the sick, disabled, the suffering, the dying, and to the person who has died, is necessary.

A person's formal or informal education, acquired through experience, must be considered. Included in this factor would be an investigation into any specialized language used by the client through education or employment. Specialized interpretations or uses of words and phrases or of foreign words or phrases are important to know. For example: the nurse needs to know how the 2-year-old shows that he needs to urinate or defecate. Failure to understand his communication of these needs may create a problem for the child where none existed before. This is particularly significant when the child is away from the home setting—as in a child health clinic, a day care center, or a pediatric unit of a general hospital. Another important facet of the educational factor is to assess the client's problem-solving ability.

As to socioeconomic status, it is important to assess the client's perception of his status. The perception and expectation of clients with varied socioeconomic backgrounds—from the deprived to the well endowed—must be considered. The impact of the client's job on his perception of himself as well as on the needs fulfilled by his job must be determined.

The assessment of growth and development should be broadened to include physical, social, intellectual, and personality elements in establishing growth and development patterns. Age, sex, and culture are inextricably bound to growth and development and may be assessed simultaneously.

To assess biologic, physical, and emotional status, the nurse needs a model of wellness to serve as a base. The model must incorporate such factors as age, sex, socioeconomic status, and culture. Models of wellness may differ for different age groups, for men and women, and for persons from varied socioeconomic and cultural backgrounds. Knowing what is expected or normal for bodily and psychic functions provides the framework within which the status of each can be assessed for a person or a family. The nurse must know what constitutes normal nutrition, fluid and electrolyte balance, oxygen demand, elimination of wastes, rest and sleep activity, hygiene, circulation, comfort (freedom from pain and discomfort), recreation and diversion, and sensory stimulation. This knowledge gives the nurse a broad framework within which to work, but is of minimal value until she assesses the normal variation for each sub-factor for a specific person. When additional data are forthcoming about this person, judgments are made from these initial data. For example: if a person's blood pressure is 110/80 mmHg, this may be considered normal. However, it may also be a sign of organic disorder in an aged person who normally has a blood pressure of 150/90 mmHg. A clear picture of what is normal for each particular person is of prime importance.

The nurse must have a knowledge of major pathologic and psychopathologic insults to the human person at various age levels, for each sex, for the major racial and cultural groups, and of those prevalent in specific geographic areas or in a certain environment. For example: structural abnormalities, malnutrition, infections, cancer, and accidents are major problems among infants and young children; for the preschooler, communicable diseases, dental caries, schizophrenia, retardation, speech defects, leukemia, and kidney infections must be considered. The older child, the adolescent, and the young adult are prone to accidents, respiratory conditions, allergies, cancer, obesity, suicide, schizophrenia, communicable diseases, behavioral problems, such as faulty eating and sleep patterns, interpersonal maladjustment, speech disorders, learning difficulties, and acne. As a person advances in age, conditions causing illness and death become more numerous. Major disabilities are related to cardiovascular-renal disease, cancer, diabetes, pneumonia and respiratory impairments, suicide, and accidents.

With a knowledge of normal human function and a working knowledge of major psychopathologic and pathophysiologic insults, symptoms of onset, causes, patterns of treatment, and outcomes, the nurse is prepared to begin the assessment phase of the nursing process. She must focus on prevention, as well as care of the sick, and rehabilitation. She continually increases her knowledge of wellness, of alterations from wellness, symptom manifestation, treatment, human reactions to illness, and qualities of coping ability, by evaluating her own actions and studying the assessment and analysis of problems presented by persons with a major disability.

When assessing a person's interactional patterns and his ability to cope with his problems, the nurse determines ways and means available to him should a crisis or stressful situation arise. Coping patterns vary greatly among individuals and within family groups. The number of variables that constitute a stress situation may determine a person's ability to cope successfully with a problem. This ability may differ from time to time and is influenced by his view as to what constitutes a stressful situation. In family settings, the ability to cope with a problem or problems may be pooled and some of the detrimental effects of a stressful situation may be offset by the strengths of individuals in the family. Interactional ability may bear on how, when, and in what manner particular basic human needs are met. This is especially true for such needs as safety, love, and esteem. It can also be true for physical needs and for adult self-fulfillment.

Considering the person's life style, his expectation of health care, his view of his own health and/or illness, and what he expects of health practitioners, the availability and accessability of human, health, and material resources, may help to determine whether he presents himself for a health status evaluation or for the diagnosis and correction of a health problem, or if therapy that is instituted will, in fact, be successful. One's life style, including the environment in which one lives and works, cannot be separated from the person if that person is to be viewed in his entirety. Failure to consider a person's life style constitutes one of the many affronts to personalization rampant in the health care system. This failure may create problems where none existed, or it may create an atmosphere wherein therapy will not be helpful. The following example will support the nurse's need to determine life-style factors, if the assessment is to designate correct and useful action.

SITUATION REPORT

Mr. Strong, a 70-year-old gentleman with swollen ankles, pain in his legs, and difficult breathing was admitted to a health care facility for diagnosis and treatment. A plan of nursing care was to be developed. This was his first hospitalization and his first evening was described as uneventful. He was given a sedative and hypnotic at 8:30 PM. At 1:30 AM, the night nurse found him walking in the hall. She intended to escort him to his room, but as she approached to take his arm, he became frightened, and quickly struck out and hit her on the lip with his hand. She became frightened; the night supervisor was called and arranged to have the night nurse's bruised lip treated. She then summoned

*the security guard who found the patient, frightened
and confused, hiding in the bathroom. He was put to
bed, and the following morning the day nurse found
him awake, upset, and worried. He told her that he
thought he hit a nurse but wasn't sure. During the
period of care, the nurse found one bit of information
about this elderly gentleman which had not been known
to nursing personnel or if it had been, it was not considered important or useful. The patient had been a
night watchman for 40 years up to the day of his admission. His sleep-awake pattern was therefore different
from that prevailing in the health care facility. He had
worked alone, policing the halls and rooms of the building at which he had been employed. He had to be on the
alert so as to protect himself against intruders. Sharing
this information with the nursing staff made quite an
impact. The nursing care plan that subsequently evolved
included efforts to help the patient reverse his day-night
pattern while he was hospitalized. He was helped to stay
awake for longer periods during the day. His medication
for sleep was changed and given to him at midnight.
Having this information on the day of admission, giving
it value, and incorporating it into the nursing care plan
might have spared the patient and night nurse an un-
pleasant experience and the negative feelings that arose
from it.*

Nursing History

A nursing history is taken to obtain needed data systematically, through a planned interview with a client. The
collection of this information, the analysis of data, designation of problems for nursing intervention, and the implementation and evaluation of this plan are the responsibility of
the professional nurse. A specific time must be designated to
obtain the history, and the place where it is to be taken—an
inner city clinic, the client's home, a hospital room, a physician's office, an industrial camp or community mental health
center—should afford privacy. The history should be taken as
soon as the nurse and client confront each other. The time
spent should be adequate to obtain as much information as
possible in an unhurried manner. Time should be given to

impart information to the client. An interview guide developed by the nurse, or by a committee of nurses, may be used initially. A number of authors have developed nursing history guides that could be useful to the beginner.[11-14] Some of these guides lend themselves to inpatient where others can be adapted for outpatient interviews. The format of the interview should vary according to the setting and services rendered and to the role of the nurse. While core data about the client as a person will always be needed, specific areas of information will differ if the nurse is admitting a woman in labor, if the client is being admitted into the health care system, or if the client is being interviewed in a self-care unit, a long-term care facility, or in his home.

In some instances, checklists and questionnaires have been devised for the convenience of the staff and to save time. Often these can be used routinely and contribute a negative factor because only items on the form are used. At times, it may be appropriate for the client to fill out information sheets. This, of course, is only appropriate if the client can read and write and if he is oriented, aware, and has the strength to do so. In any case, an interview with the nurse should verify, clarify, and yield additional information deemed necessary. The interview gives the nurse the opportunity to see the person and to use her perceptual abilities not only to obtain information but to communicate her concern, interest, and willingness to understand. It gives her the opportunity to reinforce those behaviors conducive to wellness.

The nurse should strive to develop her own format, which should allow for flexibility and adaptability with persons having a variety of problems. Eventually a specific guide may no longer be necessary. The nurse will focus on general and specific topics, making adjustments as they are needed, to obtain the data she needs to assess the client's health status and delineate his problems accurately. Making inferences about information and validating them emphasizes the nurse's desire to get an accurate picture of the client's experience and will minimize the possibility of imposing a judgment based upon inadequate information, a few symptoms, or a limited social history. This will also protect the client from becoming the recipient of stereotypes, prejudices, or generalizations inherent in the nurse.

The time spent in obtaining a nursing history is well spent; it may be a significant factor in saving time in any services or care rendered to the client. Failure to obtain data about the client before problems are assumed or solutions imposed may be more time consuming, drain the physical and emotional energy of the nurse as well as the client, and create a climate of mistrust and insecurity for him. It would add considerably to the cost of his care.

During the interview, the nurse should seek to clarify points that are not understood. She should allow the client to express himself completely and obtain a clear picture of his expectations. Should he be unable to express his needs because he is too young, too old, too sick, unconscious, or is in a life-threatening situation, a person who knows the client well should supply available information. All efforts should be made to involve the client as soon as possible and as much as possible. For example: as soon as the life-threatening situation has eased, the client should participate as much as possible. This holds true for all clients who are unable to participate temporarily or who can participate partially or only on a nonverbal level. The nurse will use her own senses to collect information as well as consult with family members, neighbors, co-workers, and other health team members during the interim in which the client cannot participate. As soon as possible, the nurse will continue with the nursing history.

Up to this point, verbal interaction between nurse and client has been emphasized. The nurse uses various communication techniques as open-end questions, and/or reflection, to facilitate communication. The selection of techniques and their appropriate use is based upon how they are used and if they facilitate exchange of data. A technique is not good or bad within itself. How appropriately it has been used and the outcome will designate its value. The nurse and client have picked up nonverbal cues that must be clarified and verified. The nurse has exercised her perceptual and observational skills to note the client's posture, facial expression, manner of dress, physical limitations such as the failure to use a hand, an arm, or a leg, to note deformities, an absence of parts, such as teeth or extremities, the presence of scars, discolorations, cuts. The nurse uses sight, hearing, touch, and smell to collect these data. (See Appendix B for a list of observations which can be made using sight, hearing, smell, and touch.)

While sight and hearing are used extensively throughout the interaction, touch can elicit data about skin temperature, muscle tension, moisture, variation in strength of extremities, swellings and masses, palpable distortions in configuration, areas of pain and tenderness, and tremors. The nurse's sense of smell can supply data relative to usual and unusual odors, pinpoint specific breath odors, such as tobacco, alcohol, mustiness, sweetness, use of chemicals—commercial mouth washes and agents that are unknown or not easily recognizable, smells which denote one's pattern of living or job, smells of wounds, particularly those infected or with decomposed or dead tissue, odors of bodily excretory products—urine, feces, vomitus, sweat, and such odors as perfumes, medicines, liniments, salves.

The nurse will measure bodily function, using palpation, observation, and measuring tools, such as thermometer, stethoscope, or sphygmomanometer, to obtain readings of body temperature, heart rate, quality and characteristics, respiratory rate, and blood pressure. Specimens such as urine, stool, vomitus, sputum, and secretions from other bodily parts, or draining wounds may be collected. Some tests can be done immediately, using chemical tapes and kits. Others must be sent to the laboratory for analysis.

The nurse could assign supportive health and nursing personnel, qualified to collect specimens and proceed with analyses, to assemble these laboratory data.

When the client feels he has had an opportunity to express his feelings, concerns, goals, desires, and expectations, and the nurse has affirmed and validated any inferences and there are no gaps in the information she needs to make a nursing diagnosis, the interview can be terminated. At this point the client can be told how these data will be used as well as the plan for continuing the interaction into the planning, implementing, and evaluating phase. The client should have felt that the nurse was interested in him as a person and that she had conveyed in her communication—both verbal and nonverbal—that she viewed him with respect and dignity. The fact that she called him by name, listened with full attention, anticipated his questions, and spoke with him rather than to him, conveys respect. She will have refrained from using language unfamiliar to him and guarded against responding to his questions in a condescending manner. If his condition was critical, with life-threatening respiratory or circulatory problems, she participated in relieving the crisis and then focused immediately on his participation. She also was attentive to the desires and concerns of persons important to the client.

During this interview, the nurse and client begin a relationship based upon trust, respect, concern, and interest. The client should feel that the nurse is truly interested in him as a person, that she is concerned about his welfare, and that she recognizes and respects him as a co-partner, designating and meeting his needs for health and nursing care.

When this nursing history interview is terminated, the client should know who the nurse is; who will be responsible for his care; that some one person knows his views, his fears, his concerns, and his expectations; that someone knows the basic human needs that he fulfills himself and those he cannot fulfill. He knows how to summon the nurse, where she will be, when and how he can communicate with her, and when she will see him again. If he is an inpatient in a health care facility, orientation to the environment and available services may be included in the interview. The nurse may consider it prudent to delegate this orientation to another member of the nursing team.

After the data are collected, the nurse seeks additional relevant data from family members, from persons accompanying the client, or from persons in the household. Other members of the health and nursing teams, significant members of the community, and available records and reports are also used to obtain data.

The nurse sorts, organizes, groups, categorizes, compares, analyzes and synthesizes the data about the client obtained up to this point. Decision making and judgment are inherent in every phase of the nursing process and are particularly significant during assessment. The nurse decides what to ask, when to ask it, and how to ask it. She decides when to listen, how to listen, and how long to listen. She uses judgment throughout the interview by focusing on some areas in depth and by passing more briefly over others. She judges when there may be more to the meaning of a topic than that which the client has told her. She summarizes all available data, then makes one or more of the following judgments:

1. No problem exists and the client's state of wellness is affirmed. Periodic reassessment of wellness will be planned, and the client will present himself for these at given intervals. The client will seek reassessment sooner if he suspects a problem.
2. No problem exists, but there is a potential problem which may be offset by giving the client information on prevention and planning for a future interview with him. It may be necessary to refer the client to another health care member.
3. A problem exists but is being handled successfully by the client and/or his family. Plans for periodic reassessment will be formulated, and the client will return for these at nonscheduled times if he thinks it necessary. The problem may be new or it may be a long-standing one. Pharmacologic and mechanical aids may be used to resolve the problem. For example: medications, crutches, hearing aids, colostomy and ileostomy appliances, prostheses.
4. A problem exists which the client needs help in handling. Providing this assistance—whether it is information, environmental, caring, socioeconomic, pharmacologic, and/or mechanical, will either resolve the problem or make it easier for the client and/or family or neighbors to handle it. Appropriate provision, including referrals to health team members and social agencies, will be planned with the client. The client, nurse, and other health team members share in implementing the plans. Implementation continues until evaluation indicates that the problem has been resolved or has decreased.
5. A problem exists which the client cannot handle at this

time and its nature prevents family and neighbors from helping him to resolve it. Health care intervention is needed. Specific members of the health care team such as the physician, nurse, dentist, psychiatrist, physiotherapist, or nutritionist may be assigned to help the client. With health care intervention (one or more members), the problem can be specifically diagnosed, treated, and resolved. An example of such a situation is dental caries.

6. A problem exists that must be studied further and diagnosed to resolve or to keep it within manageable proportions. Ambulatory and/or inpatient health and nursing services may be needed. The problem may be solved completely; for example: a foreign body or obstruction of some kind is removed. In other situations, an elevated blood sugar may be diagnosed, treated, and provisions then made for continued management on an ambulatory service.

7. A problem exists that is not incapacitating to the client at present, but to resolve it requires intervention that would render the client dependent for a specific period or indefinitely. Surgical interventions and certain medical regimens are examples. Inpatient care is generally necessary. A specific medical diagnosis may have been made before the initial nurse-client interaction. Acute care followed by extended care and/or ambulatory care may be part of the planning.

8. A problem exists which places heavy demands on the client's ability to cope with it and which the family cannot resolve; they could, however, contribute emotional support and money for intervention by members of the health care and/or nursing team. These problems may be life threatening; for example: myocardial infarction, cerebrovascular accident, diabetic acidosis, cirrhosis of the liver, bleeding peptic ulcer, drug addiction, depression. Immediate and continued intervention by members of the health care team, on an inpatient basis, is required.

9. A problem is imposed unexpectedly upon the client or his family through an accident, injury, or natural disaster, or is self-imposed (attempted suicide). The problem may or may not be a threat to life. If it is life threaten-

ing, health team members must attend to it immediately to reduce the crisis situation, if possible. If not, the crisis imposes problems upon family members. If the crisis is resolved or the situation is more incapacitating than life threatening, situations discussed in items 1 to 8 may prevail. An example would be the child who is found to have an obstruction in the respiratory tract. Removing the obstruction—a bottle top, balloon—quickly and effectively relieves the problem, with no residual disability. If the problem cannot be resolved, immediate surgical intervention may be required.

10. Problems exist that are long-term and permanent. The client is able to cope with some but not all of his problems, and others, such as family, nursing and health team members, clergy, lawyer, or social workers, may have to intervene to cope with the problem and provide care on a continuing basis. Long-term health and nursing care must be provided within the home, community health center, community mental health center, an extended care facility, or a combination of these.

Any one, or any combination, of these situations may exist for a client at one point in time, but he may experience any number of these situations in his progress to wellness. The nurse then, as noted above, designates specific problems stemming from the larger problem area.

Nursing Diagnosis

The nurse concludes the assessment phase with a nursing diagnosis.[15-18] This diagnosis specifically indicates that: (a) no problems exist which demand the intervention of the nurse or another member of the health team, or (b) the precise identification of all problems that had to be resolved so that the client could experience the wellness optimum for him. Problems will be stated in terms of client problems, and result when basic human needs are either not met or are met inadequately.

PLANNING

The planning phase begins with the nursing diagnosis. During this phase plans are made with the client to deal with his problems, as diagnosed. The purposes of the planning phase are: (a) to assign priority to the problems diagnosed; (b) to differentiate problems that could be resolved by nursing intervention, those that could be handled by the client and/or members of the family, and those that had to be referred to other members of the health team or handled in conjunction with health team members; (c) to designate specific actions, and the immediate, intermediate, and long-term goals of these actions, as well as expected behavioral outcomes for the client; and (d) to write the problems, action, and expected outcomes on the nursing care plan. The planning phase terminates with the development of the nursing care plan, which is the blueprint for action, providing direction for implementing the plan and providing the framework for evaluation.

If no problem exists and the nurse verifies the client's state of wellness, a plan for periodic reevaluation of the client's state of wellness is formulated jointly. Plans to continue wholesome living patterns will be reinforced, and specific information the client requests or needs will be given, such as: immunization, accident prevention, poison control information. Brochures may support and reinforce or expand the information. The client is requested to return immediately if symptoms appear or if he feels he has a problem. Thus in her interaction with the well client, the nurse participates with him in the assessing and planning phases, but the implementation and evaluation phases are the client's responsibility.

Ordering or Priority Setting

If specific client problems are diagnosed, effort is exerted to assign priority to each. The nurse uses her own judgment and considers the client's views in assigning priorities. Ordering or priority setting can be conveniently classified as high, medium, or low priority. As high priority problems are resolved fully or in part, the order in which remaining problems are resolved may have to be reevaluated. Problems in the medium- or low-priority category may be given a higher rating at some time. The more life threatening the problem is, the higher the priority assigned. A number of problems may be considered high-priority simultaneously, such as an obstructed airway, ineffective breathing, impaired circulation, or gross hemorrhage. It could be assumed that the nurse and the client and/or his family would generally agree about giving life-threatening problems a high priority.

Each client problem should be so classified that the integrity and unity of the human person is maintained. Again, Maslow's hierarchy can be useful in designating priority, with physical problems given priority over safety needs, then needs for love, esteem, and self-actualization. While physical needs take precedence, as soon as problems that stem from an inability to meet basic human needs at this level are diminished, high priority must be transferred to problems that arise because basic human needs in other categories have not been satisfied effectively. In some nursing situations, there may be no problems with physical needs initially, and high priority is given to needs for self-esteem. For example, the client who has a poor opinion of himself may disregard safety measures and refuse to eat. Resolving the problem with self-esteem may also solve problems in other categories that stem from the original problem area.

In all situations, the client should be closely involved in decisions setting levels of priority or order. In instances in which the nurse and the client assign different priorities to the same problem, the difference can be resolved by mutual communication of the reasons for setting a particular priority. Priorities set by the client should be considered.

Other factors that influence priorities as set for the client include the availability of personnel and resources; the cost of needed services; and the approximate time needed to resolve his problem or problems, particularly from his point of view.

Once priorities have been identified by the client and the nurse, an ordering of these priorities is established. The nurse designates possible solutions for each problem diagnosed, but solutions offered by the client should be included. The possible success of each solution to a problem is estimated, based on scientific principles and/or sound research. Variables such as age, sex, life style, education, socioeconomic, and cultural background of the client, his ability to cope with his problems, his physiologic and emotional status, as they relate and effect suggested solutions, should be considered. The nurse predicts, as accurately as possible, the consequences of each solution. Then, in cooperation with the client, she selects the solution most likely to be successful in resolving or diminishing his problem. If the client endorses the solution, his efforts and cooperation in implementing that solution will insure its success.

The solution may be multifaceted, with immediate, intermediate, and long-range implications. An immediate goal is one that can be accomplished in a short span of time. An intermediate goal can be attained over a period of time—teaching, supporting, preventing acute problems—while a long-range goal is oriented toward the future. Goals for the client include preventive and rehabilitative aspects as well as crisis or immediate aspects relative to his present wellness-illness status. For example: if the client's problem is constipation and this difficulty has been a long-standing one enhanced by the frequent use of laxatives and self-administered enemas, to relieve the condition temporarily would not resolve the problem nor would it provide long-term benefits. The client may experience immediate relief, but requires sustained relief if an impact is to be made upon the problem and if discomfort, inconvenience, and the cost of relief measures are to decrease. While the solution may be to relieve the constipation, the actions instituted may have an immediate effect—to give immediate relief by using pharmacologic or mechanical agents. Additional actions may have intermediate and long-range goals, such as developing a regimen to increase fluid intake, increase fruits and vegetables in the diet, plan specific time for defecation, and provide privacy and an unhurried atmosphere, while enemas and laxatives are gradually withdrawn. This regimen would be instituted after pathologic conditions that cause constipation, such as strictures, tumors, congenital anomalies, have been ruled out. Thus, to relieve constipation for the present would not have a lasting impact on the problem, causing the client to return repeatedly to obtain relief.

Intermediate and long-range goals that stem from solutions to the problems will be concerned with preventing complications, rehabilitation, and health instruction. Continuity of care is enhanced by this farsightedness, and the cost of health care, both in time and money, to the client and to health personnel will be considerably less. Immediate, intermediate, and long-range goals of the solutions are appropriate if the problem can be resolved and in those situations in which the problem will continue. Long-range goals may focus on preventing additional problems or preventing intensification of the present problem. This would be true, for example, when the problem is permanent blindness. Failure to designate long-term goals may mean the difference between a client who can become maximally independent as he strives toward the optimal degree of wellness for his particular problem or a client who remains dependent and therefore derives only limited joy from living because of multiple complications and problems.

When a problem that can be resolved by nursing intervention has been identified and the best solution has been selected based on the strengths and resources of the client and/or his family, the availability and competency of nursing and health personnel, and the resources available for health and nursing care, specific actions and expected outcomes for the client's problems must be designated.[19]

Problems that can be resolved by nursing intervention must be differentiated from those that not only require the attentions of a nurse but also that of one or more members of the health team, such as a physician, physical therapist, or pharmacist, and problems that can best be resolved by other members of the health team or by specific members of the community. Problems relating to spiritual or legal matters—a will, housing, job—should be referred to the appropriate person or agency. A well-designated and developed referral system should be established so that appropriate persons can be involved with a minimal loss in time, and maximum use be made of persons and agencies qualified to solve various client problems. Methods and forms are generally available for use by agency health care personnel.

Nursing Orders

The solution to any one problem may be an adaptation of a known solution or it may be designed specifically for that problem. When the solution most likely to be successful is selected, specific nurse actions designed to achieve the short-term, intermediate, and long-range goals of that solution must be delineated. These actions are also called *nursing orders*. Nursing actions must be clear, purposeful, moral, capable of being accomplished, and adapted to the particular life situation, beliefs, and expectations of the client. Since nursing action is designed to solve the problem, the outcomes expected as a result of that action should be stated in terms of the client's behavior. Only by recording the client's behaviors can the nurse judge the impact of her action. Statements of nurse behaviors can be a basis for evaluating the nurse's competency, but if the effectiveness of the care rendered is to be evaluated, expected outcomes must be stated in terms of client behaviors.

In some health care settings, established policy may dictate the kind of action to be implemented and the person who will implement that action. Policies pertaining to nursing care should be formulated with nursing personnel. Health team members may develop policies and procedures for handling particular problems or governing some particular area in a health care facility. Policies bypass thinking; the person involved in implementing a policy must know the specific circumstances under which it applies. When the situation is recognized, the policy is applied. Policies may vary from one designating the number of visitors per hospitalized client to established policies and procedures formulated in the event of cardiac arrest. They appear to be more numerous in settings where personnel tend to be less prepared. Thus, there are policies to safeguard clients. For example: a policy stating that every hospitalized client 65 years of age or over must have side rails on his bed probably resulted when it became evident that older clients often fall from their beds during their periods of hospitalization. This policy does not protect the 50-year-old with an orientation or behavior pattern that might result in a fall. Nursing judgment is needed to interpret policies and make appropriate adaptations in the best interest of the client. Policies and procedures need to be reviewed from time to time. Circumstances under which they were formulated may no longer exist and other policies may be needed. The nurse must be informed of prevailing policies, for and by whom they were instituted, allowable latitude in their interpretation, and what procedures must be followed to change the policy. The nurse is obligated to bring to the attention of appropriate persons policies potentially detrimental to clients or which are misinterpreted or overly implemented by personnel. Clear, precise policies and procedures developed for units such as coronary care, kidney dialysis, or intensive care help these facilities function quickly and smoothly. These policies also should be reviewed periodically, particularly if clients demonstrate high levels of anxiety, signs of sensory overload, or sensory or sleep deprivation. Precise data to support any request for a policy change that would improve care and enhance the individuality of the client would be helpful. All policies should be expressed in writing and dated to safeguard the nurse against pressures that perpetuate patterns of action that are custom rather than policy.

The quality and quantity of nursing actions delineated to solve a client problem and effect a specific behavioral change will be determined by the nurse's knowledge and experience. Her knowledge of biologic, physical, and behavioral sciences as well as her nursing knowledge, clinical experience, and knowledge of resources—persons, books, her ability to seek out consultation from other nurses or health team members— broadens the options, variations in actions, and the application and expectations from the actions. The nurse designates actions which will most likely effect a behavioral change and which have been approved by the client. Documenting these nurse actions—what should be done, when, and how—constitutes nursing orders.

When actions are designated for problems, according to priority or ordering, a decision is made as to who will carry out these actions, when, and how. The nurse may select those she will do for and with the client, those the client can perform for himself or which can be performed by his family without or with supervision, and those actions that can be accomplished by certain members of the nursing team. To assign the nurse who is best able to perform the nursing actions—making adaptations and modifications to suit the client, his strengths, limitations, level of wellness, illness, and personal preferences—a team conference may be appropriate for planning. It not only serves to orient nursing team members involved in the care of the client but may be useful to insure that the client's interests and preferences will be considered, his basic human needs met, and his problem solved.

It must be obvious to the reader that both the assessment and planning phase draw heavily on intellectual skills—critical thinking, decision making, judgment, observation—and interpersonal skills. The latter are used to establish rapport through verbal and nonverbal communication, including active attentive listening. Technical skills are used in both phases, but to a lesser extent than are intellectual and interpersonal skills.

During the entire planning phase, activity is directed toward the quality and quantity of nurse actions that will be needed to resolve or minimize problems. This activity effects specified behavioral change within the context of immediate, intermediate, and long-term goals, and culminates in the formulation of the nursing care plan.

Nursing Care Plan

The nursing care plan includes precise data about a specific client. These data are organized in a systematic, concise manner which facilitates overall medical and nursing goals. It clearly communicates the nature of the client's problems and the nature and relationship of related medical and nursing orders. It contains all information about the client, his preferences, his problems and the priorities assigned to each, problems and complications to be prevented, and expected outcomes with prescribed nursing actions.

The format for the nursing care plan should flow from the goals set. Space should be provided to designate client problems, solutions, nurse actions, and expected outcomes. The health care agency may have a nursing care plan form. If none is available, a nursing care plan form can be developed that would be appropriate to clients and to problems that are most likely to be seen in the health care facility. A number of authors have contributed substantially to nursing care plans and nursing care planning. [11, 12, 13, 14, 20]

A well-written nursing care plan provides a central source of information about the client with a description of his problems and a plan of action to solve them. A nursing care plan has become increasingly important with the increased number of professional and nonprofessional personnel involved in the nursing and health related services rendered to the client.

The plan is developed by the professional nurse who obtained the data for the nursing history; she is most knowledgeable about the client and has the data needed for planning effective nursing care. The plan she develops incorporates the medical care plan so that designated regimens complement rather than conflict or oppose each other. When the most knowledgeable person creates the nursing care plan, the client's individuality as a person is most likely to be enhanced. She is the one who is most likely to know the client's ability to cope with situations; thus, intervention will not be planned where none is needed and at those times when the client is coping with his problems satisfactorily. The client's right to appropriate independence, as well as to interdependence and dependence in the management of his wellness and illness is fostered.

The development of the nursing plan is, therefore, a knowledgeable, creative, and intellectual activity and should be so designed as to mark its identity explicitly, even if the client's name is omitted. When one nurse is responsible for developing and keeping the plan viable, additional data about the client obtained by other nursing and health care personnel can be directed to her. Often, important data are lost or given low priority when they are submitted to the wrong person, or the receiver places little value on the information because she has no knowledge of the client's problems or his goals.

A clearly stated nursing care plan is the most effective means of assuring the client his problems will be solved and his basic human needs fulfilled. Problems created by failing to realize some basic human need and by using verbal statements or nonverbal gestures that are depersonalizing or lower the client's self-esteem could be minimized. The drain on the time and energy of nursing personnel and the frustration and anxiety experienced by the client when he senses that the staff is not interested in him or is unaware of his needs and his preferences can be problem-solved. If the client knows the nurse is interested in him, if he knows what to expect and the person to summon, he is likely to be more relaxed and less anxious. He also is less likely to make frequent requests for errands or small duties—often only to assure himself that someone cares and knows that he exists. If they know the client's problems, his preferences, and his life style, the actions of the nursing staff will be more useful and purposeful. Time wasted through ineffective or multiple actions by many nursing personnel, because goals are lacking, communication is poor, and facts about the client are not being used properly, could be reduced substantially.

Taking the time for a nursing history, a nursing diagnosis, and a nursing care plan that includes writing orders is time well spent. Failure to take the time to assess and plan before intervening contributes to the misuse of time and wasted efforts and talents of nursing and health care personnel. The cost in economic, physical, and emotional terms can hardly be estimated. Economically and morally, the profession of nursing cannot permit this misuse of human and material resources.

Two client-nurse situations that will help to focus on these points are as follows:

SITUATION 1.

Mrs. Weak, a 48-year-old woman who was discharged after a two-week period of hospitalization was referred to a community health nurse. The referral stated that Mrs. Weak had had gallbladder surgery. Her medical diagnosis was terminal carcinoma, primary site, the gallbladder. The nurse went to the client's home to evaluate the situation; actually she should have gone to assess the client situation. Perhaps she was influenced by the fact that Mrs. Weak was terminally ill. When she went to the home and found the woman alone seated in the living room, the nurse could only recommend that she seek admission to a nursing home. The nurse was informed that Mrs. Weak's husband had been taken to the hospital with chest pain the day she was discharged. The nurse did not feel it safe for this woman to be alone. Mrs. Weak firmly refused to consider the nursing home, and the nurse's anxiety about her mounted. When the nurse returned to the community agency, she expressed her concern to her supervisor, who helped her by logically delineating the data in the situation so that a more accurate judgment could be made about Mrs. Weak being alone. To her surprise, the nurse did not know whether Mrs. Weak could walk, care for herself, or what assistance from family and neighbors, if any, was available to her. Did Mrs. Weak know how to summon help for herself in case of an emergency? After a thorough assessment, it was found that Mrs. Weak could manage very well by herself and actually had little disability, considering that she had a terminal illness. An effective assessment preceded the development of a plan of care acceptable to Mrs. Weak. It was realistic and focused on the wellness she experienced as well as her illness.

In another situation, automatic actions based on a specific condition rather than the condition within the context of the client's total situation caused the client to refuse nursing care.

SITUATION 2.

Mrs. Wise was a 40-year-old woman who was admitted with a diagnosis of anemia. She was ambulatory, and the medical plan was designed to find the cause and type of anemia as well as to determine appropriate treatment. Mrs. Wise was a career woman who had a responsible job. While assisting with the physical examination on the day Mrs. Wise was admitted to the health care facility, the nurse noted that the client had a colostomy. Without obtaining further information from Mrs. Wise, the nurse planned to irrigate the colostomy the following day. She attempted to do so, but Mrs. Wise promptly and clearly refused her help. The nurse felt that the client had rejected her, for she thought she was being helpful. She had overlooked the fact that Mrs. Wise had had the colostomy for 14 years and had established effective regulation without irrigation, with minimal care, and without assistance. Also, during these 14 years, Mrs. Wise had never disclosed to anyone but her husband that she had a colostomy. Had the nurse assessed the client's problem and taken a nursing history, she would not have been rejected and would have used her time and energy more purposefully, directing her actions to include the problem that brought the client to the health care facility—anemia.

Planning has two additional dimensions: horizontal and vertical. Horizontal planning has been discussed up to this point as: problem—solution—goals (immediate, intermediate, long-range)—nurse actions. The additional dimension involves vertical planning, which fosters the logical progression of nurse actions and has its greatest impact when the nurse and client interact on a continuing basis throughout a 24-hour-period. Vertical planning includes timing specific actions, paying special attention to basic human needs and the client's circadian rhythms. For example: if the nurse is required to perform numerous actions and there are accompanying actions by other members of the health team, such as a physical therapist, occupational therapist, medical technologist, physician, actions should be planned to permit undisturbed periods of sleep and undisturbed meals. Not to include these considerations during the planning phase may cause problems for the client and divert some of the energy he needs to cope with the task at hand away from fostering an improved state of health. Thus, the time factor is a major consideration in planning. It involves not only the amount of time required for and when nursing actions will take place, but the biologic timing of the client, which must be known and preserved.

Once developed, the nursing care plan is implemented. At this point, the plan should not be considered a finished product. It is merely a guide to actions and must be kept viable by additions and changes based on the client's problems, on resolving these problems, and on collecting data continuously as nurse and client get to know and trust each other.

The format of the nursing care plan should be such that it is easy to use and contains enough space to record everything that needs to be written down. While brevity and clarity are characteristics of a useful nursing care plan, its use will be diminished considerably if brevity becomes the exclusive goal. The development of the nursing care plan is the nurse's privilege and is, in fact, a creative, purposeful, intellectual activity. It is an expression of a nurse's knowledge, her ability, and her focus on the client. It will also serve as the model for all actions initiated by other members of the nursing team. Thus, the nurse contributes to the effectiveness and goal-direction of others—all of which benefits the client.

Every effort should be made to develop a method of displaying and storing the nursing care plan so that it is readily available to the nurse when she needs it. No one should have to wait to review the plan because someone else is using the folder that contains it. Space should be provided so that changes and dates can be filled in without erasing. For study and research, the nursing care plan and how it evolved should be preserved, since it contains first-hand data about persons, their problems, solutions to these problems, and goals that may be useful in developing a nursing science.

It is interesting to note that Bertha Harmer made similar statements in 1926 in her book *Methods and Principles of Teaching the Principles and Practice of Nursing*. She suggested that nurses develop a written program of nursing care and that these programs be kept and filed under a classification of diseases. She felt that nurses would collect a mass of information about nursing specific persons and about nursing in general. Organized knowledge would be available in a form which permits the nurse to go back and check her work, to note progress in content and method and ". . . to compare facts presented for the study of a great many cases of the same class, and of different classes, and to select facts common to all cases of the same class; in other words, to formulate principles, to organize knowledge—the process of making knowledge, which is science."[21]

Also, the plan can be used as a model for the care of other persons with similar problems, with a similar ability to cope with problems, or it can serve as a point of self-improvement for the nurse as well as for all members of the nursing team.

Sharing the nursing care plan with nursing and appropriate health team members fosters a better understanding of the client, and the efforts of all health and nursing personnel are more likely to complement each other. Each team member will find that she can function in her role more effectively and successfully when the roles of her associates are clarified. Health team members should be encouraged to utilize the nursing care plan as a resource.

The planning phase ends when the nursing care plan has been designed and developed. This plan is an effective medium for transmitting information for planned care in that all team members can accurately perceive and implement the care intended. It should be designed so that it can be utilized quickly and all nurse actions are meaningful and directed toward resolving the client's problems.

In some situations, client problems, particularly those that are critical in nature, may be preplanned for use within the framework of the nursing process. Preplanning involves the use of nursing or problem-solving processes to develop plans of action when time is important and life may depend upon a predetermined plan of action. An example of such preplanning would be actions to be taken in case of fire. Available data about fires, how they start, various types of fires, combatting various types of fires—electrical, chemical, combustability of materials, level of vulnerability of a particular setting, fire regulations, materials available to extinguish fires, techniques for safety of personnel and clients, and methods of prevention should be sought. In addition to literature and manuals, a specialist in fire fighting should be sought for consultation. A plan could be drawn up by nursing and health team members, clients, and other interested persons, then tested for accuracy and efficiency—including dissemination of the plan, instructing personnel on their roles, testing equipment. A periodic review to reinforce the plan should be scheduled. Thus, as soon as the nurse assesses the fire, the plan indicated by the situation is implemented. The applicability and effectiveness of the plan can only be evaluated after it has been used. Preplanning may include all members of the nursing team in a particular setting, health team members, and citizens. Other situations in which preplanning is valuable include such crises as cardiac arrest; mass disasters, such as floods and earthquakes; drownings; explosions; emergency treatment for accidents (poisonings, burns). The more intense the crisis and the greater the immediate threat to life, the less time there is for thinking and problem-solving and therefore the more important preplanning becomes. The plan is revised as new knowledge of how different crises should be handled becomes known. Thus, there is less time between assessment and implementation phases. When the crisis has passed or diminished, the usual problem-solving methods prevail.

In addition to preplanning by health and nursing team members and citizens, the nurse may find it necessary to preplan a selected number of problems to enhance the safety, security, and life of the client, and which could be used until the problem is relieved or its intensity and immediacy diminishes. For example: if the nurse is working in a school setting and among the students there are a few with epilepsy, she may preplan the care they should receive for a seizure. This preplanning involves collecting a great deal of data about the client's pattern and manifestations of convulsion; the presence or absence of an aura; the client's method of handling himself before the onset; the characteristics and effects of the convulsion; data from the literature about convulsive sei-

zures; identifying problems associated with convulsive sei-
zures (falls); known methods of promoting safety and minimizing injury during or after a seizure; identifying persons
likely to be involved, such as teachers and classmates; ramifi-
cations for the client when a seizure occurs during a swim
class, in the science laboratory, in the lecture hall; formulating a plan of action in the event of a seizure and communicating that plan among teachers, friends, the client, or selected classmates who may become involved. Suggestions shared
by these persons should be incorporated into the plan. Once
the plan is implemented, it should be evaluated. Other plans
might be devised by the nurse, as she needs them; for example: what to do in the event of sudden death (in whatever
setting this may occur), choking, obstructed airway, hemorrhage, to mention a few.

Preplanning may be appropriate for anticipated crises and
problems, where thinking and planning time is limited and
where immediate action is necessary to enhance the client's
safety. Preplanning focuses on an event and is often heavily
technical. Continued preplanning beyond the selected crisis,
for more than "just in case", or outside the framework of the
nursing care plan defeats its purpose. Preplanning should be
used within the various phases of the nursing process, and
incorporated into a client-centered, goal-directed framework.
Excessive, exclusive, or inappropriate use may be dehumaniz-
ing and depersonalizing, focusing on an event or problem
rather than on the client or focusing on one problem to the
exclusion of others. It can add a measure of confidence to
the nurse and security for the client if she knows what to do
in an emergency. Preplanning may be strategic in that it may
help the nurse prevent a situation, and the plans should be
shared with nursing and health team members, family members, and the client, if appropriate.

IMPLEMENTING

Once the nursing care plan has been developed, the implementation phase begins. Depending upon the nature of the
problem and the condition, ability, and resources of the cli-

ent as well as the nature of the action planned, the client or his family, the nurse and client, the nurse alone, or nursing team members who are to act and function under the nurse's supervision may implement the nursing plan. Implementation also may be accomplished by the nurse, assisted by nursing team members, or in cooperation with health team members. Any combination of or all of these situations may prevail. In other words, in any one situation, some planned actions may be accomplished by the client, some by the nurse, and others by nursing team members. In other instances, only the client may be involved. This is particularly true if the client is well and prevention is the goal. The client may be able to continue wholesome health practices or new health practices in place of faulty ones. Some or many care measures may also be performed by the client's family, not only for clients who are homebound, but also for inpatients in health care facilities.

The implementation phase of the nursing process draws heavily upon the intellectual, interpersonal, and technical skills of the nurse. Decision making, observation, and communication are significant skills, enhancing the success of action. These skills are utilized with the client, nursing team members, and health team members. While the focus is action, this action is intellectual, interpersonal, and technical in nature.

With the nursing care plan as the blueprint and immediate, intermediate, and long-range goals firmly in focus, actions are put into practice. During this phase, the viability of the nursing care plan is tested. The plan is not carried out blindly, with all thinking and decision making accomplished during the two previous phases.

The nurse continues to collect data about the client as a person, his condition, his problems, his reactions, his feelings. Additional information continues to be gleaned from other nursing and health care personnel, and from family, neighbors, teachers, and records.

The success or failure of the nursing care plan depends upon the nurse's intellectual, interpersonal, and technical ability. This includes her ability to judge the value of new data that become available to her during implementation, and her innovative and creative ability in making adaptations to compensate for unique characteristics—physical, emotional, cultural, and spiritual—that become known to her during her interaction with the client. She must have the ability to react to verbal and nonverbal cues, validating inferences based on observation. Paramount during the interaction is her acceptance of herself as a person, and confidence in her ability to perform the independent nursing functions inherent in the planned action, recognizing those which are dependent and in which she contributes to fulfilling the medical care plan. She must have a realistic understanding of herself, recognizing and accepting her strengths and limitations; be convinced of her own personal worth and find meaning in her life; meet her own basic human needs reasonably well, so that she can, with willingness and joy, give of herself to another—her strength, her courage, her faith in the competency of the client, her value for life, her knowledge, her skill, and her time during the interim when these might be needed by another. She must feel comfortable being herself—authentically herself. She needs to feel secure and adequate in her relations with others. If her needs are satisfied and she can control her own thoughts, feelings, and actions, she will be able to focus on the thoughts, feelings, and needs of another in a wholesome comfortable manner. While the nurse meets many of her needs outside the nurse-client interaction, her needs for recognition, monetary compensation, creative expression, and self-fulfillment are satisfied in her role as nurse through her interactions with clients, their families, co-workers, and colleagues.

The more wholesome her view of herself as a person and the stronger her philosophy of life, the less likely the client will experience depersonalizing encounters with the nurse.

The following situation, as told by Nurse B, illustrates an inadequate and inappropriate interaction during the implementation phase:

When 65-year-old Mrs. Brave was admitted to the hospital on an ambulance litter, it was evident that she needed an admission bath. I, Nurse B, was asked to help Nurse A. Mrs. Brave moaned but did not talk. She lay in the fetal position, on her right side. She could not or would not change her position. Nurse A reacted roughly, making comments about how dirty the patient's family was. The poor lady, I am almost positive, must have heard what Nurse A was saying. At this point I believe Mrs. Brave was frightened and, perhaps angry, so that she became increasingly uncooperative. I tried to talk to Mrs. Brave to reassure her that she had nothing to fear from me and that I was not going to be unnecessarily rough with her. I said nothing about her odor; Nurse A referred to it almost constantly. I tried to encourage Mrs. Brave to help with the bath and extend her extremities. With two nurses attending her, it must have been very confusing to Mrs. Brave; she did not know to whom she should respond. Nurse A did not cover her very well while bathing her, and as I tried to cover Mrs. Brave she grabbed the covering and drew it tightly about her. Apparently Mrs. Brave had been sick for a while at home and had no one to care for her except her husband.

The nurse should feel confident, comfortable, and satisfied in relating to clients. If she does so, she will not use the client, her co-workers and colleagues, or the setting to satisfy her own personal needs. While assessment and planning require these same qualities in the nurse, the implementation phase tests her endurace, her love, her intellectual ability, and her interpersonal and technical skills.

The amount of time spent with the client varies significantly, ranging from a short to a prolonged interaction. This encounter could be in terms of minutes and hours per day to daily, weekly, monthly, or yearly continuation of the relationship; the interaction may be continuing or intermittent. Interaction should be planned precisely by the nurse and client, with allowances made for the unexpected.

It is strategic that each interaction be goal-directed and purposeful. An atmosphere of intellectual and interpersonal "thereness" should prevail. In other words, the interaction demands alert, observant, attentive behavior by the nurse. In this atmosphere, the nurse conveys her concern for the client, her interest in helping him achieve the wellness optimum for himself. In her manner of speech, her tone of voice, her gestures, and mannerisms, she imparts her views of this person as one who has dignity and value. This means conveying dignity and value even though the client may not feel, look, or smell good, or if he acts, looks, or thinks differently.

In the client's presence, the nurse uses her perceptual skills to their fullest. As she looks at the client, maintaining eye contact as much as is comfortable, she observes his situation—his posture, appearance, and actions, his immediate environment, and the presence of other persons. She may initiate conversation or allow the client to do so. The client is given the opportunity to direct the conversation and initiate topics of interest to him. The nurse actively listens to what he is saying, indicating by nods or short statements that she understands. She asks for clarification if she does not understand and helps the client focus on a topic if he has difficulty doing so. She adjusts and adapts her manner and the content of her communication with the client when the situation is such that verbal expression is difficult, temporarily not possible (client has a tracheostomy), or is permanently impossible. The nurse must be able to judge when it is necessary to listen more patiently, when an interpreter is needed, when mechanical devices such as paper and pencil are needed, when hand signals can be used. The nurse and client will also need to know when verbal communication is not necessary, silence is appropriate, touch is useful and appropriate as well as when and where it should not be used, or when words are conveying a message different from the nonverbal message coming through. The nurse judges how to word her statements and questions in a manner that will elicit responses within the client's capabilities (physical, emotional, social, educational), and uses repetition, as needed, without demeaning or demoralizing the client. If the nurse cannot understand the client's message, she freely admits this and seeks ways or persons who could enhance her understanding.

The nurse is fully aware of the need to communicate with the client who does not respond in the usual and expected manner. Talking to the infant or to the comatose or unconscious client is important, not only from the standpoint of conveying a message, but to maintain as much sensory integrity and contact as possible. The verbal as well as the accompanying nonverbal message may be received, even though the receiver is unable to return verbal messages. The nurse can meet needs for safety, security, love, and esteem by talking to the client, by her manner, or her voice, particularly if she holds the client's hand, feels his brow, or supports a shoulder. Further, very young or very old clients who are isolated, or who become disoriented, may feel alone or abandoned if human contacts are limited or task-centered. It is extremely important to prevent sensory deprivation for these clients.

The nurse may find that the client needs her full attention and she will choose to sit with him in full view, yet with the privacy of their interaction protected. At other times, she may find that while bathing or feeding the client opportunity will be available for conversation. Since the nurse has considerable data about the person, she will be able to use them to explore or suggest topics. She may plan a caring activity, using this activity as a vehicle to foster conversation. The nurse will judge when technical activity will enhance the client's safety and security more than verbal assurances. Thus, by viewing action in terms of the goals of nursing care, based on client problems, the nurse's focus on achieving a goal is facilitated, often meeting needs on several levels simultaneously by a particular action. For example: relieving dyspnea has physical as well as emotional implications for the client. If the nurse does not perceive or respond to the client's dyspneic state his anxiety may increase, adding additional stress to his respiratory reserve.

When the purpose of the nurse-client interaction is to perform a technical action, the success of the nurse's activity can be heightened if she focuses on the recipient's immediate needs as well as on the technical procedure itself. The client is entitled to an explanation of the action, his role and expected behavior during the action, the expected results of the action, the type of equipment, solution, etc., the discomforts to be anticipated, the position to be maintained, and how much privacy will be afforded. The client not only is informed, but the message he receives loudly and clearly is that the nurse is sensitive to his needs, knows the technical aspects and expectations of the procedures, and considers him a person. The equipment should be assembled outside the immediate environment, if possible, particularly when discomfort is associated with the technical action, the requisite equipment is not prepackaged, considerable time is needed to prepare the equipment, or the nurse needs to take more time to organize and familiarize herself with the use of the equipment and the procedural method, or needs to consult someone about the technical aspects of its use or procedural method. If the technical aspects are to be performed by or in cooperation with another member of the health team, a mutual understanding of the role of each person (nurse, health professional, client) and the requisites for the procedure should be established in advance. The client's preparation and participation should be clarified before the technical action is initiated.

The nurse continually uses decision-making skills, judging when the procedural method and the timing of the technical action must be modified, or consultation with or assistance from other persons is necessary to assure a safe, effective action.

In each contact with the client, she not only focuses on the purpose or goal of the interaction but continually expands her perceptual ability to obtain data about the client that would indicate the planned action is correct. She seeks data that would indicate other problems due to unmet or poorly met basic human needs. She continually reviews the client's reaction to her thoughts and actions, for he quickly picks up discrepancies between verbal expressions of interest and concern and actual practice. When the client is not called by his name, the nurse fails to look at him, uses a brusque manner, is impatient, rough, or focuses on a body part or piece of equipment rather than on him, her disinterest in him as a person is clearly evident.

If another member of the nursing team assists the nurse with planned actions, special attention must be paid to the client-centered focus. Conversation between or among nursing personnel in the presence of the client should focus on and include him. Social conversation or conversation pertaining to other clients, or about nursing and health care personnel has no place in the immediate client setting. Further, the client quickly picks up the nurse's and her assistant's lack of interest, attention, and concern. The impact may be quite serious if the client's ability to cope with the situation is strained, his concept of himself is low, and if he is apt to misinterpret motives. While light conversation may be very appropriate and may serve as needed diversion, it should include the client and be of interest to him.

> *Lois Lawst, a 10-year-old girl with diabetes, was in the treatment room waiting for the nurse who was to teach her how to administer insulin. Two other nurses and two nursing students had accompanied the client to the treatment room after requesting her permission to observe her progress. During the waiting period, some questions were directed toward the young girl and, initially, the conversation included her. Shortly, however, the conversation drifted away from the client, and the four nurses soon became deeply involved in a personal conversation that portrayed a socioeconomic status far different from that of the 10-year old. She sat alone and was temporarily forgotten. Only when the expected nurse arrived was attention directed back to the client. Lois refused to give herself insulin that day.*

As the nurse proceeds to implement the nursing care plan, she learns more about the person, his reactions, his feelings, his strengths, his limitations, his coping ability, his preferences, his satisfactions, and his dissatisfactions. She learns his response to planned nurse actions, additional ways available to him and to the nurse to perform actions, the need for additional actions, and any untoward response to the planned actions. These data are synthesized and utilized to further develop the nursing care plan and are the basis for recording data about the client on appropriate nursing records.

If the nurse finds that some or selected actions should and could be performed safely by other members of the nursing team, she should delegate these actions. She knows the capabilities of nursing team members, and should also know the responsibilities of persons with a particular title as well as those who have a specific role. She needs to know the strengths and limitations of the individuals in these roles. She should focus on selecting the most appropriate person to perform a specific action for the client. The person so designated should have as much information about the client as she needs so that her actions are truly effective and the nursing team member is able to perform in an informed manner. Thus, delegated activities are part of the whole focus of action and contribute purposefully to immediate, intermediate, and long-range goals of care. The person performing the delegated tasks is responsible for her own acts and is expected to report the outcome in terms of the client. The nurse supervises the performance of supportive nursing personnel.[22-25] Data about the client obtained by team members should be communicated to the nurse responsible for his care and for implementing the nursing care plan. If more than one nurse is involved in the client's care, particularly in inpatient settings, written and verbal reports concerning the client as well as an up-to-date nursing care plan are needed to insure continuity and goal-direction. If each nurse is responsible for the client's care, each should participate in changes needed to keep the nursing care plan viable. If conflict arises relative to the interpretation of goals specific to the action to be taken by the nurse, the priority of action to meet the desired goal, or client responses differing at different times of the day, a conference should be planned with the nurses involved and with the client to resolve it. This does not necessarily mean that two different means could not be used to achieve the same end because the views, knowledge, or experiences of the nurses involved differed. Resolution is needed only when conflict involves a goal or priority opposing that planned with the client.

In designating the *who* in terms of planned nurse action, the nurse may feel that she is the best person to perform the action at a particular time. She may require assistance and will decide on who, the number, and kind of assistance she needs. She may delegate selected nurse actions to other nursing personnel. This pattern may vary from time to time, from day to day, and even from moment to moment—always dictated by behavioral changes in the client, available nurse manpower, and the coping ability of the client and his family.

She gives care if she is the best prepared person to implement the particular action from an intellectual, inter-personal, and/or technical standpoint. She may find that her performance of a particular action will serve as a vehicle or means to meet safety, love, and needs for esteem. She may wish to use her presence—her thereness—to give the client an opportunity to express himself and to share his doubts, fears, and anxieties.

Just as the nurse's philosophy, education, and experience influenced the type and character of nursing actions she designed to meet problems, so will these significantly affect implementing the actions. Her emphasis, her focus, and her creativity will be affected by her own strengths, limitations, prejudices, stereotypes, her knowledge of human behavior, the strength of her convictions, her ability to handle human closeness, and her ability to use herself therapeutically. Her willingness to share her knowledge and give of herself, as well as her knowledge of her intellectual, emotional, social, and spiritual boundaries, will influence what the nurse will do, can do, and knows enough not to do.

Gentleness, sureness, and strength can be conveyed by the nurse, not only to alleviate associated discomfort, embarrassment, or frustration accompanying the problem, but to actually meet some basic human needs—love and safety.

If other persons are involved in the client's care, the nursing care plan gives direction to the actions of nursing and health care personnel. But the actions and activities of these persons need to be coordinated to make them person-centered and to make certain that vertical planning is implemented. Coordination takes into account who is doing what and when. This assures that actions are taken and that the client's biologic rhythms and his situation are benefited rather than overwhelmed. It is possible that an action may be ineffective simply because it is poorly timed, or is done in conjunction with other actions which may conflict or interfere with each other. For example: a health professional enters the room to treat a client with a poor appetite just as he begins to eat. Or she plans a care activity just as a visitor enters the room of a lonely client. Persons involved in activities with a client may influence the performance of a specific action because of the variation in approach. For example: the manner in which a client is helped out of bed, how he is supported, which side of the bed is used to get him out of it, whether he is allowed to dangle before he gets up may influence his desire to get out of bed, the amount of time he spends out of bed, and what he does when he is out of bed.

Due to the client's response during implementation, priorities may have to be reassigned, and reassessing and replanning will then be required. Nursing judgment is needed to know what to do with data, the additional data needed, what the data mean, whether a new nursing diagnosis is needed, and what the plan of action should be.

Thus, the implementation process, while it does have an action focus, includes assessing, planning, and evaluating activities by the nurse. The actions of implementation performed with and for the client could include: inserting, withdrawing, turning, cleansing, rubbing, massaging, flexing, irrigating, manipulating, teaching, exercising, offering, awakening, cuddling, holding, drying, applying, communicating, administering, influencing, altering, relieving, supporting, cooling, warming, providing, accompanying, sitting with, listening, walking, moving, touching, soothing, pulling, pushing, straightening, twisting, wrapping, folding, flexing, to mention a few. Strategic to these actions are those related to assessing, planning, and evaluating, which complement the action implemented. These actions are needed to resolve, dissolve, and diminish the client's problem.

The actions may be independent or dependent functions of the nurse. The latter relate to carrying out doctor's orders for drugs and treatment, which are part of the medical care plan. Dependent functioning does not imply following orders blindly and without question. Critical thinking and sound judgment must be exercised to make decisions about what, when, how much, and in what manner. For example: specific nurse action planned to relieve pain should follow a careful assessment of physiologic manifestations of the pain; its location, quality, and character; severity; what the pain being experienced means to the client; and other factors. The nurse needs to know the pattern of the pain, verbal and nonverbal evidences, and gestures. The nurse may be able to utilize pharmacologic measures and/or manipulate the client by changing his position, removing wrinkles or restrictions, and by actions that influence his behavioral response to pain. McCaffery[26] summarized the physiologic and physical factors influencing the client's sensation of pain and his behavior associated with it as: (a) neurophysiologic processes underlying the sensation of pain, duration and intensity of pain, alterations in the level of consciousness, cutaneous versus visceral sites of pain, environmental conditions, sensory restriction, physical strain and fatigue; (b) cultural aspects, including sociocultural group membership, age, sex, religion, body part involved in the pain, roles ascribed to members of the health team; and (c) psychologic factors, including emotionally traumatic life experiences, secondary gains of the client's complaint of pain, personal past experience with pain, knowledge, understanding, and cognitive level, powerlessness, attitude and feeling of others, perceptual dominance of pain.[26] Thus, the client's pain involves more than automatically administering a prescribed analgesic when he states that he is in pain.

The implementation phase concludes when the nurse's actions are completed and she has recorded the results of actions and the client's reaction to them. Recording these actions and reactions is an important function of the nurse. The quality of the recording about the client and what the nurse chooses to document give direct evidence of the status of goal-achievement and individual client reactions, and designates the status of and the direction for continued problem-solving. Placing a low value on recording, or insufficient or inappropriate recording, is an affront to the client and demonstrates the nurse's limitations. Automatic notations or general statements give little or no indication of the client's individuality, his problem, and his reactions to the planned action. The recordings are related to the problem; they describe the nurse's actions and the results, and include additional data. The written report of nursing care given serves to direct continuing action. Communication—oral and written—associated with the nursing history, nursing diagnosis, nursing orders and actions, client actions and reactions, should be given a high priority by the nurse. Her recording should reflect the client's unique situation and should be identified easily by the quality of their content. The recording should contain the information needed to give a profile of the client. Rules that set limits on what and how much should be recorded and that have only one basis—supposedly to save time—can be a waste of time. The nurse must decide what to write, how much to write, when to write, and that which is important. Writing associated with the development of the nursing history, nursing care plans, and recordings about an action performed is a professional not a clerical activity. Nor should it be delegated to persons who are not prepared to assume this important professional responsibility. Specific recording of data certainly may be delegated, but not the nursing history, the nursing care plan, or recording significant data about the client that stems from implementing the plan. Recordings are more frequent when the client's behavior changes rapidly. If these changes occur slowly and are infrequent, there will be less to record but the information will not lose its significance. When recordings become copious or their use is minimized because one does not have the time to review them, the information should be summarized periodically in coordination and in conjunction with the nursing care plan. It would be helpful to index recordings of client progress. The process of indexing would be based upon significant experiences or stages in the resolution of a problem, and would also be useful for nursing care plans. If plans have been developed over long periods of time, a new or revised nursing care plan should be developed. All previous plans or additions to it should be retained as long as the client has problems that have not been resolved or which are being dealt with but cannot be resolved. Plans developed with persons who are well or for whom health prevention and maintenance are major goals will be reactivated, as needed, for reassessment. These plans and records should be retained for evaluative purposes and future planning.

Thus, the implementation phase of the nursing process includes nurse actions determined by the nursing care plan.

The nurse continues to focus on the client, conveying, through her intellectual, interpersonal, and technical skills, that he is indeed worthy of her respect and is imbued with dignity. Nurse actions are based upon scientific rationale and directed toward promoting a suitable internal and external environment in which wellness is enhanced and illness diminished. Factors in the external environment include influencing significant legislative actions, particularly those related to health and environment. Available resources and their appropriate use are inherent in the implementation phase. The appropriateness and direction of the nurse's action(s) are determined by the client's behavioral change in the direction of goal achievement. The direction and amount of change is evaluated.

EVALUATING

Evaluation, the fourth component of the nursing process, follows the implementation of actions designated in the nursing care plan. Evaluation is always in terms of how the client is expected to respond to the planned action. Since specific nurse actions were planned to solve client problems, any judgment about how these problems are being resolved should originate with the client.

The nursing care plan contains the framework for evaluation. The impact of all intellectual, interpersonal, and technical actions upon the client and the changes these produce are the focus of evaluation.

While elements of evaluation, like those of assessment and planning, are concurrent and recurrent with other components, evaluating the effect of actions during and after the implementation phase determines the client's response and the extent to which immediate, intermediate, and long-range goals are achieved. The evaluation must continue in a purposeful, goal-directed manner. For example: if relief of pain is to be expected from implementing the nurse action, the results would be known within a short period of time. The client would tell the nurse that his pain was or was not relieved. The nurse could compare the client's premedication behavior, noting posture, facial expression, pulse and respiratory rates, color of a part, his ability to focus on other topics and other persons rather than on the pain. There would be substantial behavioral evidence that would indicate the client's pain was fully relieved and the nurse actions had brought about that relief; or the nurse could conclude that no pain relief or limited pain relief was obtained and her actions had been ineffective or partially effective.

Evaluation is the natural intellectual activity completing the process phases because it indicates the degree to which the nursing diagnosis and nursing actions have been correct. By evaluating nursing actions the nurse demonstrates that she accepts responsibility for these actions and shows her interest and involvement in enhancing the effectiveness of actions directed toward solving the client's problems. It also demonstrates that the actions are person-centered and there is less likelihood a nurse action will be continued if it is not helpful.

Evaluation will also pinpoint omissions during the assessment, planning, and implementation phases. In any given client situation, it is possible that some problems may be resolved at different time intervals. Since evaluation will be in terms of immediate, intermediate, and long-range goals, the evaluation process is continued until these goals are realized. The outcome of the evaluation may indicate the care planned must be reassessed, replanned, modified, and the revised plan implemented and evaluated. Thus, the nursing process is a continuing cycle.

The nurse and client are the agents of evaluation. Other persons, such as the client's family, nursing personnel, and health team personnel, may also be involved. Based upon the behavioral expectations of the client relative to the mutually agreed upon immediate, intermediate, and long-range goals, measurement data are collected so that value judgments can be made. A number of measuring devices and methods are available to obtain these data. These data include: temperature recording, pulse rate, blood pressure recording, apex rate, electrocardiogram and electroencephalogram recordings, and a gamut of physiologic analyses, such as urinalysis, blood sugar, blood urea nitrogen, cholesterol. The condition and situation of the client—his posture, appearance, color, level of orientation and statements—made by his family and significant others knowledgeable about his situation—should be used by the nurse in her evaluation. The nurse uses her senses to collect data; she utilizes communication techniques to elicit subjective data (questioning the client about dizziness and nausea), makes inferences and validates them, and makes a decision about the client's behavioral response.

The outcome of evaluation may be any one or a combination of the following:

1. The client responded as he had been expected to and his problem is resolved. No further nursing action is needed. Followup may be planned to determine that his problem has not recurred. An appointment may be made for a future date to reaffirm the client's problem-free status.
2. Behavioral manifestations of the client's situation indicate his problem has not been resolved but evidence demonstrates immediate goals but not intermediate and long-range goals have been achieved. The nature of the client's problem is such that complete resolution, if it is possible, will be slow. The nurse action is then geared to intermediate and long-range goals. These goals include preventing anticipated and possible problems. Reevaluation will continue.
3. Behavioral manifestations of the client are similar to those evidenced during the assessment phase. Little or no evidence that his problem has been resolved is available. Immediate goals have not been realized; there may or may not be evidence that intermediate or long-range goals may begin to be realized. Anticipated and possible problems may or may not have been prevented. Reassessment with replanning is needed.
4. Behavioral manifestations indicate new problems. Assessment, planning, and implementing a plan of action to resolve this problem are in order. Planning action to resolve the new problem must be coordinated with the planning for the previously diagnosed problems. Evaluation will follow implementation.

If the nurse has used the logical, goal-directed problem-solving approach of the nursing process, evaluation should indicate a high level of success. Involving the client and his family in the nursing process contributes to this success. The likelihood that any or all of the client's problems will not be resolved is decreased.

While the profession of nursing is directing its efforts toward developing standards for the practice of nursing, these standards are broadly stated and are applicable to all clients who enter the health care system, particularly the nursing subsystem. Standards of nursing practice are stated in terms of a systematic, goal-directed, problem-solving approach. The profession fulfills its obligations to provide and improve nursing practice by developing these standards, which are now recognized by nurse practitioners. The standards convey to the citizenry a model of service that can be expected from members of the profession and their assistants. The nurse actions directed toward resolving client problems are guided by these standards, and action is measured and compared with the standards. Evaluation of nurse actions purposely directed toward the client's problem, as included in the nursing care plan, is applicable to a specific client.

As in all other phases, the client is involved in evaluation. While specific nurse actions may be found to be highly effective, moderately or minimally effective, or ineffective, these conclusions can only be reached after the degree to which the client's problem has been resolved is evaluated, based on the behavioral manifestations he demonstrates. Judgment during other phases may have resulted in immediate reassessment and replanning. But only during the evaluation phase is a comprehensive appraisal of goal achievement—immediate, intermediate, long-range—made. After client behavior is evaluated, the quality of nursing care and its impact upon the client's health status is determined.

Some of the questions the nurse can ask during this evaluation phase are: What was the expected client behavior? Was the expected behavior realistic, accurate? What data supported the judgment that the behavior was realistic and accurate? What behavior was manifested? What tools or instruments were utilized to obtain the data? What observable data were collected? What judgments were made concerning these data? What subjective data were collected and documented? Were data synthesized and compared before the value judgment was made? Does the client agree with the judgment? Do other members of the nursing team and health team concur with the value judgment?

What goals—immediate, intermediate, long-range—have been or are being met? If goals have been met, what are the plans to periodically reassess and maintain a problem-free status?

What factors influenced goal attainment? What factors influenced the limited or lack of goal achievement? Were these factors internal and/or external to the client/his family, the nurse, nursing team members, health team members, other persons such as friends, neighbors, co-workers? What factors were related to the setting in which the nursing care took place—the home, the clinic, industry, a health care facility? Were environmental, socioeconomic, cultural, or religious factors involved?

What additional data are needed? How should they be obtained? From whom should they be obtained—the client, his family and associates, the nurse, doctor, pharmacist, teacher, or employer? Are data needed from one or all of these sources?

Were the nursing diagnosis, nursing orders, and nursing care plan accurate and realistic? Was the plan of action accurate, but the action ineffective because it was not carried out accurately, was inept, or it did not consider the client as a person? Was there input from the client? If not, why not? Was the nurse action accomplished by the wrong member of the nursing team? Was it a nurse action at all or should it have been accomplished by the client and/or his family members, or a member of the health team?

Are some problems partially resolved? How is this partial response determined? Is it due to factors in the client's internal or external environment? Could the problem have been resolved completely if additional data had been sought or an alternative solution tried? Was the assessment complete? Was the nursing diagnosis correct? Did the problem resolve itself despite omissions in assessment, planning, and implementation? What contributed to this resolution?

If the client's behavioral manifestations indicate his problem was not resolved, what were the reasons? Were there physiologic, psychologic, intellectual, socioeconomic, cultural, and religious reasons for the lack of resolution? What external factors are influencing this failure to solve his problem? Do the nursing care and medical care plans conflict rather than complement each other? Is there a lack of resources (human, financial, technical)? Is there a permanent handicap, an incomplete understanding of the problem and its impact?

Has the situation been labeled a problem when it is not a problem? Do the client and the nurse want to relinquish the problem? If nurse action was deemed appropriate but the results of the action were ineffective, what was the reason? Was timing incorrect? Did the appropriate member of the nursing team implement the action? Was consideration given to the age, sex, developmental level, and role of the client? Is the limitation due to the nurse's intellectual, interpersonal, and/or technical skills or to those of a team member?

Was communication effective? Was the message received identical to that sent? Did feedback verify the accuracy of the message?

Did the client suffer an affront to his feelings as a person—failure to identify him by name, focusing on a part rather than the whole person, attending to equipment rather than the client, ignoring persons significant to the client and their participation in his care? Was recognition given to the psychologic, emotional, religious, cultural, and socioeconomic influences inherent in the client situation and accompanying implementation of nurse actions?

Was the intent of the goals clear—immediate, intermediate, and long-range? Are new problems evident? Are they related to other unresolved client problems? Are they unrelated? What data are available about the new problem? Is the problem known to the client? What is his reaction? Is the new problem the result of new pathology, changed socioeconomic status? Is it the result of nearsightedness in anticipating problems? Is it the result of a change in the client's role, his diminished ability to cope with his situation, or a change in body image? Are there changes within the family system?

Are there previous problems that have not been dealt with? How have long-range plans influenced these problems? Have they been realistic? Have these plans and related actions made an impact?

Were the immediate, intermediate, and long-range goals geared to preventing disease and maintaining health as well as to sickness care, if needed?

Were the nursing actions based on principles from the physical, biologic and behavioral sciences? Was the nurse action stifled by a rigid policy interpretation, failure to accept the fact that there are independent functions of the nurse?

When the data for evaluation are collected, analyzed, and synthesized a new picture emerges. The nursing care plan may continue as designed or it may need to be revised partially or completely. Additions may be made or alternative action selected. The client situation may indicate a transfer to a health care facility (from a general hospital to a nursing home or vice versa) or even a transfer to another unit of the same health care facility (from intensive care to a surgical unit).

Changes in the client situation or location within the health care system may involve other health professionals. The balance of action geared toward maintaining wellness, preventing illness, giving care during sickness, or fostering rehabilitation may show a directional shift toward the client or toward the nurse.

Once the new status (direction of change and progress toward goal achievement) is designated, based upon the evaluation, either the problem is resolved and no further nurse action is needed or new priorities are set and goals determined. Modification is incorporated in the evaluation phase and follows it. Modification results in reprocessing activity, feeding back to assessment for reassessment, and continuing the cycle of each phase. The cyclic process is continued as long as it is needed; in other words, as long as there are goals to be achieved or until the client completes his life span. If the goal that is to be achieved is to maintain the client's well status, periodic reassessment may continue for an unlimited time span. The nurse-client relationship may reflect periodicity rather than a continuous hour-by-hour interaction.

In viewing the use of the nursing process with a client longitudinally, the time interval of nurse-client interactions may demonstrate periodic, continuous, or any combination of periodic and continuous interactions, as evidenced by the client's wellness-illness profile over a span of years.

The act of evaluating may be strengthened and clarified by the following examples. An interaction was heard one morning in the nurses' station of a coronary care unit. Three nurses had the following conversation:

Nurse A: *(leafing through the client's chart). I think we should talk about Mr. Klotz. He's the client with a myocardial infarction, who came in two nights ago. This morning it was the same thing again. Complaints and more complaints. He says he can't sleep with a light on; the night nurse is too noisy; he is awakened when he just about dozes off, and the aide always bumps his bed when she goes in to do something.*
Nurse B: *What does Mr. Klotz expect in the coronary care unit? He is not the only one here. Last night there was a cardiac arrest, so naturally there would be a lot more excitement. He isn't even as sick as some of the other patients are. And the lights aren't bright. They are dimmed after 8:00. We could tell the aide not to be so clumsy. I think we should spend time talking about the sicker clients or taking care of clients.*
Nurse C: *Mr. Klotz should give his complaints to the night nurse where they belong.*
Nurse A: *(leafing through the client's chart) I disagree! Mr. Klotz may really be saying that he is very frightened of the night. Maybe he thinks he will die. And look at this! Did you notice that his pulse is higher at bedtime and during the early morning hours than it is during the day? This is documented by the monitor strip on the nurse's notes. His respirations are increased, too, and he*

is perspiring and pale. When I first see him in the morning he looks anxious. His anxiety seems to be having an affect on his cardiovascular system.

Nurse B: *That's interesting! I hadn't noticed this relationship. Maybe he is telling us something and we almost missed the message.*

Nurse C: *Yes, maybe we should ask the night nurse to join our conference so we could pool our observations and plan an approach to verify if Mr. Klotz is anxious and why. Then maybe we could help him.*

This example points up the use of specific measures to verify behavioral change.

The nurse concluded that she had adequately taught an expectant mother to bathe an infant when she observed the woman do so effectively.

The nurse was present when 20-year-old Mrs. Noo bathed an infant during a prenatal class demonstration period. When the nurse observed the client bathing her own infant during a postnatal visit to her home, Mrs. Noo demonstrated the ability to follow through safely and effectively during the bath. She had assembled all necessary items, and handled the infant firmly, yet gently and lovingly. Mrs. Noo reported what she knew and what additional information she needed. The nurse had specific data upon which to judge that a specific goal had been achieved. These data were specific behaviors demonstrated by Mrs. Noo, as observed by the nurse.

While on a home visit to assess the needs of a diabetic teenager, the nurse noted that the teenager's mother seemed worried and preoccupied. Validating her observation, the nurse found that Mrs. Frite, a 43-year-old widow and mother of three teenagers was most fearful of her own safety. She told the nurse that her mother had died of cancer of the cervix a year ago and her oldest sister was to have a hysterectomy for a cervical malignancy. Though Mrs. Frite expressed her fear of cancer, she refused any suggestion that she have a pelvic examination and a cytologic smear. If the expected behavior resulting from the nurse's action to relieve this fear of cancer was that Mrs. Frite would accept this advice, make an appointment with a gynecologist, and keep the appointment, it would have been specific be-

havioral evidence that the nurse's goals had been realized. The immediate goal was to give Mrs. Frite an opportunity to verbally express her fears of cancer and a cytologic smear, provide specific information about the smear, and assess the availability of a gynecologist in her area. Within two weeks, Mrs. Frite did follow the nurse's suggestion. Both examinations were negative for pathology, and Mrs. Frite was very relieved.

If the client has difficulty remaining oriented due to sensory deprivation, behavioral evidence within the client must be sought to demonstrate whether the deprivation was relieved. By comparing the client's behavioral profile before and after nursing action, needed data are obtained to make an evaluative judgment. The basis of sensory deprivation may be factors within the client. He may have a sensory deficit—unable to see, hear, or speak. He may be very young or very old; there may be pathophysiologic and psychopathologic reasons. He may be isolated from the mainstream of activity due to disease or therapy (staphylococcal infection, radiation treatment), or by geographic location. He may lack appeal; he may not look good, smell good, or have wholesome habits. He may have no relatives or friends; he may be unconscious, nonverbal, and withdrawn. If the problem were diagnosed and a series of nurse actions were planned to relieve the deprivation, evidence of increased orientation, cerebration, and sociability would be some of the behaviors the nurse would expect to see in the client. Of course, behavioral expectations would be those of which the client would be capable. Behavioral manifestations of lessened sensory deprivation for the unconscious client would need to be specified and observed.

If the client is expected to verbally express who he is, where he is, plan what he wants to do and then do it, or plan and know when and why he cannot follow through, the nurse will have a series of behaviors that designate a decrease in sensory deprivation and an increase in sensory input. Expecting the client to demonstrate that he is oriented in a way in which he was not capable at any time previously would result in failure to achieve a goal. For example: if a child is disoriented, expecting him to tell time and know the date may be beyond that which he is able to accomplish, considering his age and level of growth and development.

Nurses have supplied calendars and clocks; these are particularly needed if the client is in a room that does not have a window. A radio is helpful since time checks, weather reports, news events, as well as a variety of voice tones or music may stimulate the client in whom sensory deprivation is a problem. These aids are especially useful for the unconscious or blind person, and serve as adjuncts to human interaction on the verbal and nonverbal level.

The nurse will seek evidence that the client can recognize familiar and significant persons and things. She can observe the number of human contacts the client has and the quality of the interaction. Does anyone speak to the client or touch him? Does he experience variations in sensation, such as coolness, warmth, softness, roughness, smoothness?

What are the sounds, smells, sights, colors, temperature of the environment? What are the furnishings of the environment? What sensory stimulation is there for the client? Is he an active or passive recipient of this stimulation? Does he attempt sensory stimulation himself?

Is the client lethargic, unresponsive, irritable, despairing? Does he complain about limited human contacts? Is there a clock or a calendar he can see, is there a radio or television set in his room and is one or the other turned on? If the client is unconscious, does the nurse talk to him and tell him what she does when she lifts his leg or his arm or elevates the bed? Does she tell him the water is cold, warm, or if compresses are placed on his body? Does she tell him the time of day, day of the week, month of the year? Does the client hear various voice tones—masculine, feminine, loud, soft? These might be some of the questions that must be answered to evaluate changes in client responses, using the initial assessment as a baseline. The results may indicate less sensory deprivation, indicating that the nursing actions planned should be continued. Modification in terms of the kind of nursing action, the person doing the action, the intensity and timing of action, increasing the length of human contact, changing the quality of the contact, increasing the number of persons involved, may be necessary.

If the client is a child and excessive crying was diagnosed as a lack of need fulfillment, then crying should decrease after nurse actions planned to fulfill physiologic, safety, and love needs have been implemented. The actual amount of time spent in crying, the character of the cry, the amount of playful activity, evidence of contentment, improved appetite, and increased weight would be observed, recorded, and used to judge that the child's needs were being fulfilled. Nurse actions would be considered appropriate, based on the behavioral change noted in the client.

It is expected that if the nursing process is the key to solving these problems affecting the client's wellness or illness, its use should be highly effective. Supporting the degree to which success was expected is the fact that the nursing process is systematic, logical, and goal-directed, focusing on the client and his situation. The client is considered the nurse's partner throughout the phases of the process. In instances where goals have not been fully achieved and when a judgment has been made that a particular nurse action or series of nurse actions had little or no effect upon the problem for which it was planned, as demonstrated by client behavior, the nurse looks for the reason.

Sources for reasons why predicted outcomes were not realized include: the client, the nurse, other persons of significant importance to the client, nursing staff members, and health team members.

Concerning the client, possible causes include sharing inaccuracies, insufficient information, or withholding important data about self and situation. Causes for failures to realize goals can include an increase in pathophysiology and/or psychopathology, allergic manifestations, a drain on the client's expected ability to cope with his problem due to multiple influencing variables acting simultaneously. Unrealistic expectations of one's self and predicament, loss of self-esteem, loss of job, inadequate finances, untoward reaction to therapeutic agents—chemical, mechanical, pharmacologic—a lack of or an insufficient opportunity to participate in diagnosing problems and planning strategies, failure to seek immediate attention for high priority problems, a lack of interest in and attention to intermediate and long-range goals, and planned strategies and goals that have not been accepted are other reasons.

If the nurse is the source, reasons the client's problem has not been resolved may include overlooking data; assigning high or low priorities inappropriately; a failure to validate a hunch or inference; a lack of knowledge about the client's situation, particularly socioeconomic, cultural, and religious; failure to recognize intellectual, interpersonal, and technical limitations; failure to use intellectual, interpersonal, and technical strengths; inappropriate delegation of nurse actions to nursing team members; failure to consider the medical plan when formulating the nursing care plan; limited sharing of important information about the client with health team members; failure to consider the value of input from family members, employers, or teachers; excessive focus on dependent functions; inadequate fulfillment of independent nursing functions; deficiencies in taking a nursing history; failure to involve the client in planning; failure to recognize client strengths and his need for independence within the limits of his wellness or illness; ineffective and/or infrequent communication; failure to consider others significant to the client; and failure to recognize the impact the nurse makes upon others.

For nursing team members, possible reasons contributing to ineffective goal achievement may be insufficient information about the client and his problem, his expectations, or his goals; failure to convey important data about the client to the nurse who is responsible for the care plan; interpersonal affronts to the client as a person—not calling him by name; failure to insure his privacy and that of his messages; conversing in his presence without including him; failure to record important data as intake-output or changes in quality and rate of pulse; giving information about the client to a nurse not knowledgeable about the client; focusing on things rather than the client; being noisy, loud, insensitive, and forceful or domineering.

Concerning the significant others of the client, some of the reasons goals are not achieved are: they are not available or are not interested in the client; his problem, the solution, and expected behavioral change are not understood; the client has a limited ability to cope with his problem; fears and anxieties exist about self and client; they fail to see that a problem exists or resources—financial, physical and emotional energy, intellectual endowment—are limited; lack of transportation; and moral, cultural, and religious influences.

Health team members may be responsible for the failure to achieve the goals planned for the client. Reasons for failures in these cases might include a conflict of goals for the client, failure to see the impact of the focus upon a part of the client rather than the whole, inability to function as a team member, failure to see value in a nursing care plan, limited experience in communicating with members of the nursing team and other health team members, focus on technical aspects of contribution to the exclusion of the interpersonal component, and acts of depersonalizing the client.

Another facet of evaluation that has been developed in recent years is the nursing audit. *Audit* usually suggests an inspection or review of records or accounts to insure honesty and accuracy in business transactions over a particular period of time. *Nursing audit* suggests, too, an inspection or review of some type of transaction. Potential areas of nursing that can be audited are: nursing care plans, resulting client care, and a retrospective type in which the client's legal record of care is audited. A nursing audit is a review, by a nurse, of the client's care or his records to determine the extent to which that care and/or records meet established standards.

Auditing care plans developed for a client assumes that the client's status has been assessed, a nursing history has been initiated, a nursing diagnosis has been made, and nursing orders have been written. The recorded nursing care plans can be audited periodically by nurses who are less familiar with the client. The advantage of this type of audit is that it is probably a more objective audit to determine gaps in the plan or to raise questions about areas of care that should be pursued, or areas of the plan that can be approached in another way.

The client's care can be audited by observing him when that care has been completed. A semicomatose person in a hospital can be observed for such aspects of care as body position, body cleanliness, status of the environment, apparent comfort. An ambulatory amputee in a clinic can be observed to detect the correct use of body mechanics, the care given to the body area near the prosthesis, and exercising techniques. A diabetic can be observed in his own home as he administers insulin to himself to determine how well he understands the instruction given him about insulin administration.

Records tell the auditor that data have been documented; to be certain of the quality of care that has been given, the most economic, effective, and direct way to audit this information is to observe the client. Auditing the care given to him is a certain and sure way to determine the extent to which that care has met established standards. The results of the audit can have direct implications for the client under care here and now.

Following the care of any client, some type of documentation is done on a legal record; the specific type of record depends on the setting in which the care is provided. A review of these legal records is the nursing audit performed most frequently. It is a client-centered activity and is a form of hindsight or retrospective evaluation. Phaneuf[27] developed the nursing audit process which is applicable to a variety of settings, and which has as its theoretic framework the independent and dependent functions of nursing. She developed this process to determine the extent to which nursing care has measured up to the specified objectives; it is not designed to evaluate care while it is being given, nor is it designed to be used to evaluate the nurse's performance.[27]

The persons responsible for the nursing audit are the professional nurses who can function as individual auditors or as a group of auditors. They may be associated closely with the client, be completely unfamiliar with the client, or the group may be composed of some nurses who know and some who do not know the client. The first task the auditors must accomplish is to establish standards against which their observations will be measured. While several nurses may be responsible for developing these standards, performing the audit or aspects of it can be delegated to various members of the group.

The frequency with which audits are taken can be determined by the group, according to the type of client whose care is to be audited. The records of a critically ill person in a hospital will have to be audited more frequently than those of a person in a clinic. The care of chronically ill persons in a nursing home can be audited more regularly and less frequently than that of clients in a facility designed for the acutely ill. Important factors in the conduct of the audit are that nurses should be convinced of its value, should develop standards and auditing instruments appropriate to clients for whom they are responsible, and they should be motivated to continue to improve the auditing techniques for their own satisfaction and especially for the continued improvement of the care given to the client.

The audit contributes to a systematic method for evaluating client care and assigning a qualitative judgment to the care and services received by a client. The nursing audit serves to pursue excellence and to contribute to the nurse's moral and legal accountability for the service she renders.

The nursing audit can not only contribute to an improved quality of nursing care, but can also influence the total health care system. It can contribute to better communication among and collaboration with nursing and health team members. The results of the audit should be shared with all persons concerned with client care. This openness, coupled with a knowledge of the goals of the auditing process, is strategic if the nursing care rendered is to be enhanced continuously and the quality of person-centered health care increased. It may provide data needed to effect required changes in the health care system.

Thus, the fourth component of the nursing process, evaluation, the framework for which has been prescribed, stems from the nursing care plan. Evaluation is always expressed in terms of achieving expected behavioral manifestations within the client. The entire focus of the nursing process is goal-directed. It is systematically geared to solve diagnosed client problems by prescribing specific nurse actions which would most successfully induce a specific behavioral effect that would denote the client's problem had been resolved.

Evaluation aids the nurse and client to determine problems that have been resolved, those that need to be reprocessed (which includes reassessment and replanning), and the diagnosis of new problems.

The need for research and for testing solutions to client problems is heavily supported through the use of the nursing process. Data about the client, gleaned through the process, can be used in nursing research.

REFERENCES

1. Barrett-Lennard G T: Significant aspects of a helping relationship. Mental Health (Canada) Special Suppl 47:1-5, 1965
2. Maslow A H: Motivation and Personality. New York, Harper and Brothers, 1954
3. Erikson E H: Childhood and Society. New York, WW Norton and Co, 1963, pp 247-274
4. Black K: Assessing patient needs, The Nursing Process. Edited by H Yura, M Walsh. Washington, DC, Catholic University of America Press, 1967, pp 1-20
5. Frankl V: Man's Search for Meaning. New York, Washington Square Press, 1963
6. Brown M, Fowler G: Psychodynamic Nursing. Philadelphia, WB Saunders Co, 1971, pp 21-23
7. Family Coping Index, Developed by Johns Hopkins School of Hygiene and Public Health and Richmond Instructive Visiting Nurse Association—City Health Department, Nursing Service (Richmond-Hopkins Cooperative Nursing Study), Directed by RB Freeman, 1964
8. Levine M: Adaptation and assessment: a rationale for nursing intervention. Am J Nurs 66:2450-2453
9. Brown E: Newer Dimensions of Patient Care: Patients as People, Part 3. New York, Russell Sage Foundation, 1964
10. Duvall E M: Family Development. Philadelphia, JB Lippincott Co, 1971
11. Mayers M: A Systematic Approach to the Nursing Care Plan. New York, Appleton-Century-Crofts, 1972
12. Smith D M: A clinical nursing tool. Am J Nurs 68:2384-2388, 1968

13. Lewis L: Planning Patient Care. Dubuque, Iowa, WM C Brown Co, 1970, pp 35-62; 57-62
14. Little D, Carnevali D: Nursing Care Planning. JB Lippincott Co, 1969
15. Rothberg J S: Why nursing diagnosis? Am J Nurs 67:1040-1042
16. Durand M, Prince R: Nursing diagnosis: process and decision. Nurs Forum 5:50-64, 1966
17. Chambers W: Nursing diagnosis. Am J Nurs 62:102-104
18. Komorita N I: Nursing diagnosis. Am J Nurs 63:83-86
19. Smith D M: Writing objectives as a nursing practice skill. Am J Nurs 71:319-320
20. Johnson M, Davis M, Bilitch M: Problem-solving in Nursing Practice. Dubuque, Iowa, Wm C Brown Co, 1970
21. Harmer B: Methods and Principles of Teaching the Principles and Practice of Nursing. New York, Macmillan Co, 1926
22. Kron T: The Management of Patient Care. Philadelphia, WB Saunders Company, 1971
23. Douglass L, Bevis E O: Team Leadership in Action. St. Louis, CV Mosby Co, 1970
24. Lambertsen E C: Nursing definition and philosophy precede nursing goal development. Mod Hosp 103-136, 1964
25. Yura H, Walsh M B: Super-vision. Supervisor Nurse 2:18-36,1971
26. McCaffery M: Nursing Management of the Patient with Pain. Philadelphia, J B Lippincott Co, 1972, pp 27-65
27. Phaneuf M: The Nursing Audit. New York, Appleton-Century-Crofts, 1972

chapter four

Application of the Nursing Process

The nursing process can be applied in a variety of settings; it is flexible and adaptable, permitting the nurse to use her judgment and creativity in caring for the client in an organized, orderly, and systematic manner.

A number of situations are presented to illustrate: (a) the variety of clinical and environmental settings in which the nursing process can be utilized, and (b) the variety of ways in which the nursing process can be used. Eight situations have been selected for presentation. A few show how the process was used after initial attempts failed to achieve the goals set for the client. One situation is presented in the first person—the nurse involved in caring for a terminally ill person reports her experience. Other situations are presented in the third person—the nurse reports her use of the nursing process to assist in resolving the client's problems.

There is no stereotyped, *one-way-only* to proceed through the phases of the process, nor is there a definite pattern to follow in moving back and forth among and between the different phases. These are factors that are determined according to the needs of the client in each situation, and the abilities of the individual nurse. Some situations deal with several facets of client care, others deal with a limited number of problem areas.

The never-ending challenge of coping with the many parameters of human behavior constantly stimulate and motivate nurses to improve their methods of client care. Some comments appear after the facts about each situation are presented. These are only a few of the possible comments that can be made. The reader, especially the learner, is encouraged to provide additional dimensions to the recorded comments.

SITUATION:
MRS. ROSS IN A MILITARY HOSPITAL*

I said "Hello" to Mrs. Ross over a new, hand-breathing machine and she showed me how it was used. We said "Goodbye" three months later. Some of the things that occurred between the "Hello" and "Goodbye" I want to share with you. Particular emphasis will be focused on her pain and the consequences of pain.

"How well she explained the use of the machine," I thought. With several more inhalations and exhalations she completed her task. She leaned back in bed, savoring the momentary comfort it provided. Looking at me with warm brown eyes she asked: "Why haven't you been around before? I like your smile. It makes me feel good." Without waiting for a reply, her eyes sought those of the head nurse and said: "Captain Thomas makes over me and spoils me—I love it." Captain Thomas laughed and said: "You're easy to spoil." We continued to chat for a few more minutes and then I left her room. I did not realize then that this was the first of many times I'd be seeing and working with this lady.

When we returned to the nursing station, Captain Thomas, the head nurse, told me more about Mrs. Ross, a widow of some fifteen years. Her work in public services, until she became ill, was performed in Europe. She knew her job, every facet of it. Her illness began

From LTC Madelaine Bader, ANC. Journal of Thanatology, Vol. II, No. 2, 1973. Courtesy of the author and Health Sciences Publishing Corporation.

approximately nine months ago, when she developed constant right flank pain and intermittent gross hematuria. At that time, excretory urogram, cystograms, and cystoscopy were within normal limits. Because of her persistent symptoms, subsequent excretory urograms were performed which showed progressive decreased function on the right side, with normal cystoscopy examination and normal bilateral retrograde ureterograms. Finally, because symptoms continued to persist, all tests were again repeated. An associated progressive problem of hypertension, requiring medication of hydrodiuril and reserpine, evidenced intermittent exacerbations. Mrs. Ross was transferred from Europe to the United States in December for further evaluation. Captain Thomas told me that Mrs. Ross intended to return to work as soon as possible. Illness, said she, was her enemy and she did not tolerate ill health with any degree of equanimity. She was a strikingly handsome woman, with lovely white hair that was ever so slightly waved. Her attitude was regal, yet warm and responsive. Although sixty-one she appeared to be in her early fifties. In December, she weighed 133 pounds. When I met her in March, she had lost twenty-five pounds. She carried her 5'6" height gracefully. Every movement was executed with poise that completely lacked artificiality— even when she became quite ill, this quality never left her.

I must back up a bit and let you know how I first became involved with Mrs. Ross. Every fourth or fifth weekend, I, as well as other clinical chiefs, represent the Chief Nurse in her absence. One of our duties is to make rounds throughout the hospital. It was while making rounds on the urology unit that I met Mrs. Ross.

Previous to our actual meeting, I had heard Mrs. Ross' name mentioned quite often during morning report in the chief nurses' office. Since admission to Walter Reed General Hospital, she had undergone surgery for removal of her right kidney. During surgery, Mrs. Ross had a cardiac arrest, was resuscitated, and surgery was completed. The pathology report subsequently revealed adenocarcinoma with involvement of the right adrenal and vena cava. Two days after surgery, Mrs. Ross' vital signs were stable. The major problem, at that time, seemed to indicate possible renal failure. Several days later, hourly urine output had decreased markedly and Mrs. Ross was transferred from the intensive care unit to the renal unit. She required dialysis therapy for the next three days until urinary output could again be maintained by the patient. During her stay on the renal unit, morning reports indicated that Mrs. Ross was often observed crying or making cryptic comments about the patient with whom she shared the room. She wanted the patient moved to another area as she felt she needed to be alone to get the rest she required. Consistent remarks made in morning report were how "anxious" this lady appeared and how nursing staff was becoming increasingly more perplexed and frustrated over her apparent "unreasonable" demands or responses to any information or requests made of her.

My thoughts, after hearing repeated reports of Mrs. Ross' behavior and the vivid descriptions rendered by nurses reporting her condition, conjured forth a mental image of the usual stereotype—a rather cantankerous, fault-finding, demanding lady whose life style probably was in keeping with her present behavior and who no doubt was the proud possessor of three heads—all monsters.

I could scarcely believe that the Mrs. Ross I had met could be the same Mrs. Ross. I felt compelled to check with the head nurse to discover if the person was indeed she. Captain Thomas confirmed my query. "Yes, it's the same Mrs. Ross. She was transferred back to us yesterday. She's really happy to be back. I think when she saw patients receiving dialysis treatment she may well have had visions that her remaining life might consist of the same kinds of therapy." (Some days later this assumption was confirmed by Mrs. Ross as she shared, with me, some of the stresses patients could do without.)

Several busy weeks passed and I only vaguely wondered how Mrs. Ross was doing. One Monday morning I heard Captain Thomas' voice over the phone saying: "Hi, Colonel Bader, I think we could use some help with Mrs. Ross. I understand you are one of the founders of a project that's designed to help us work more effectively with terminally ill patients and with their families."*

---

*PROJECT CAM (Crisis Awareness and Management) a project founded by a nurse and social worker to meet needs of terminally ill patients and their families as well as others who may be in crisis from lesser manifestations of loss, i.e., limb, organ, role, or relationship. Teaching seminars are conducted with interdisciplinary participants, designed to assist them in dealing with their own feelings about death; to increase their awareness and sensitivity so they would become more effective in meeting the needs of terminally ill patients and their families. Upon requests from units, we go to the unit and assist staff members in problem-solving. Guidelines and approaches are suggested which they might utilize in meeting the needs of the patient and his family.

"That's right, Captain Thomas. You mentioned Mrs. Ross...." "Yes, the doctors feel her prognosis is grave. Metastasis has begun and her condition is such that they feel the only care that can now be given will be of a supportive type."

When I asked for more information about Mrs. Ross, Captain Thomas poured out a multitude of facts and feelings. Mrs. Ross' daughters were here. The doctors had · informed them of their mother's condition and prognosis. She felt both daughters accepted the news, but Sandy, the married daughter who had just arrived from Texas, appeared to be angry and unable to release any of her anger. Kitty, the single daughter who had been with her mother off and on since admission, appeared concerned with the ways she could help her mother during this critical period. I learned from Captain Thomas that she had told the daughters about me and they expressed a desire to meet me. I arranged with Captain Thomas to meet with the daughters the following day. We scheduled a meeting with staff members for Thursday. Captain Thomas indicated that Dr. Lyons, the resident working with Mrs. Ross, planned to attend the meeting.

Thursday I was on the unit a few minutes early. Captain Thomas introduced me to Dr. Lyons, while other members of the staff brought chairs into the combination doctor-secretary office which would serve as our conference room. I met the other staff members, and added to the introduction Captain Thomas gave me by briefly explaining how the meeting came about and what I knew thus far about Mrs. Ross. I asked the staff members how I might be of assistance to them. They indicated their concern that Mrs. Ross, to the best of their knowledge, had not been informed of the seriousness of her condition. They felt they were in a bind, not knowing what to say or do for Mrs. Ross. Their anger was directed towards Dr. Doe who had complete charge of her case. Dr. Lyons commented that Dr. Doe could not bring himself to tell Mrs. Ross about her prognosis, even when she asked. He and Dr. Doe had discussed "leveling" with her many times. Dr. Lyons felt Dr. Doe should tell her about her condition when she asks, without taking all her hope away. Dr. Doe apparently vascillates between telling her or keeping it from her, using as an argument that he really wasn't quite convinced the cancer had metastases—besides she never "really" asked him what was wrong with her. Staff members remarked that Dr. Doe has recently been seeing Mrs. Ross less frequently and stays only a short time. When he visits he seemed always accompanied by other doctors, and they wondered if this indicated his reluctance to be alone with her, for fear of the questions she might ask him. Staff members wanted to know how they should respond to Mrs. Ross if she asked them: "Am I going to die?" I wondered aloud if she had asked any of them that question. Captain Thomas was the only one that replied affirmatively: "She asked me. This was the other day when she was so wretched after repeated episodes of nausea and vomiting." She said: "Things look serious don't they?" "She waited for my answer and I just looked at her, nodded my head and touched her hand. She sort of sighed quietly and requested to see the legal officer. She wanted to make a statement donating her body, in case of death, to Walter Reed General Hospital."

We discussed how staff members might react if Mrs. Ross had posed this question to them. Some staff members indicated they would not be able to deal with such an inquiry, and besides "she has never given me the slightest hint she thought she was going to die."

The need to deny operates within personnel as well as within the patient. If the patient senses in personnel denial of their terminality he will not attempt to bridge that gap. However, if the patient senses that personnel are willing to deal openly and honestly with him, such as Mrs. Ross sensed from Captain Thomas, the question will be asked.

I shared with staff members the times I became disappointed with certain patients over their apparent reluctance to move towards acceptance of their illness. Only after reflection about our interactions was I able to acknowledge that it was due to my lack of readiness, in most instances, to deal with the subject of death. Each time, the patient would be quick to perceive my reluctance and quickly changed the subject to a neutral topic. Only after I recognized and worked through the reasons for my unreadiness, was I able to again confront the patient and be able to help him.

Sharing these experiences with staff members seemed to strike a response in them as they slowly recalled times when the patient gave them "cues" and they "tuned out." We should not assume that the pa-

tient has been told or has not been told about his condition. We need to take our cues from the patient and
proceed from there, continually following the patient's
pace. What the patient needed to deny yesterday, he
may be ready to deal with today.

The remainder of the conference concentrated on
identifying Mrs. Ross' needs and how staff members
could assist in meeting her needs. One need, manifest to
all staff members, was to leave the hospital and stay in
Texas with Sandy, her eldest daughter. Staff members
felt this could be her "unfinished business" and that
Sandy was the daughter she needed to communicate
with openly in the short time remaining. Kitty, Mrs.
Ross had indicated, would be alright—she had her own
internal resources and she did not have to worry about
her. How this need might be met posed formidable
problems to the staff. Mrs. Ross had been hampered all
week by progressive nausea and vomiting. How could
she be released to visit her daughter if the nausea and
vomiting persisted? Dr. Lyons indicated he planned on
inserting a nasogastric tube for draining that afternoon,
as well as obtain another GI series to ascertain what
might be causing Mrs. Ross' difficulty. They also shared
with others certain facts about Mrs. Ross—her need to
be as independent as possible. They recognized she
would request help if needed, but counted on them to
be in the room during the times she would attempt to
bathe herself, or get in or out of bed.

The conference ended with staff members determined to meet Mrs. Ross' need to get home to Texas
and spend her last few days with her daughter—even if
they had to take her to the airport themselves and accompany her to Texas!

During the next few days, Mrs. Ross responded
dramatically to tube drainage, resuming all intake with
minimal distress. It was during this time that Mrs. Ross
showed evidence of increasing discomfort. The area of
discomfort was always the same, to the right of the
abdominal midline, radiating to spine. She remarked
that she no longer was ever free from pain. She did not
like to receive pain medication for it seemed to make
her "foggy," and she either slept a great deal or, if
awake, was unable to think clearly about matters significant to her. Her ability to communicate meaning-
fully with others, she felt, was markedly reduced at
these times and she freely admitted how frightening
such experiences were to her.

One day, about a week later, Mrs. Ross remarked to me rather casually, while rubbing her abdomen: "Dr. Lyons seems to think this mass I feel is malignant—Dr. Cairns (another resident) seems to think so too—Dr. Doe is the only one who won't say either way." She looked at me and smiled wanly. Her gaze never left my face. "What do you think the mass is, Mrs. Ross?" "Well, I really think it is malignant—of course I hope Dr. Doe is right when he says it may be from surgical trauma, but I really think it's not." Her hand kept rubbing her abdomen and her face reflected both anguish and pain.

The pain. What could be done about her unrelenting pain. Right now she was sleeping a good deal of the day and most of the night. She remarked that she was unable to do the things she felt she wanted to do because of the drug's "foggy" effect. Yet the current drugs, Demerol and Phenergan, did not relieve her pain. I reviewed her orders and noted she was presently receiving the following medications: Compazine, 10 mg intramuscularly, every 6 hours or as needed for pain; Seconal, 100 mg intramuscularly for sleep, as needed; Tigan suppository, one as needed for nausea; Talwin, one tablet orally every 3 hours or as needed for pain; Demerol, 75 mg intramuscularly, every 4 hours, or as needed for pain; Phenergan, 25 mg intramuscularly, every 4 hours or as needed for pain. I wondered what the chances might be of titrating medications that would relieve her pain, yet keep her mentally alert. I discussed this possibility with Captain Thomas, and described some of the successes we had on other units when the patients became involved in the decision of scheduling their medication. Captain Thomas felt Dr. Doe would be agreeable to such a venture, and planned to talk with him in the morning.

The next day Captain Thomas called and asked me to stop by the unit if I had a moment. When I entered the nursing station, she showed me Mrs. Ross' order sheet signed by Drs. Doe and Lyons. It read: Patient's pain medication is being timed and tested for best results according to her expressed desires. She may receive: Demerol, 25 to 100 mg orally, as needed for pain; Dilaudid, 2 mg orally or intramuscularly, as needed for pain; Percodan tablets, one or two, orally or as needed for pain; Talwin, 50 mg tablets, one or two orally for pain, as needed; Talwin, 30 to 60 mg intramuscularly, as needed for pain; Phenergan, 25 to 50 mg orally or intramuscularly with any of the above medications as

*needed; Seconal, 100 mg intramuscularly, for sleep, as
needed. Drs. Doe and Lyons had stopped by Mrs. Ross'
room to briefly explain the new orders. They told her
the nurses would fill her in on the details of the new
regimen.*

*Armed with enthusiasm, expectation, and knowl-
edge of the arsenal of medications which could be used
to alleviate Mrs. Ross' pain, Captain Thomas and I entered her room to explain her role in this new under-
taking.*

*At first she listened rather passively as we explained
the list of medications available to her whenever she
expressed her need for them. We captured her undivided
attention, however, when we told her we needed her to
tell us how effective the drug was that she had requested . . . that we also needed to know any drugs that
she had received during this hospitalization that seemed
to be more helpful in controlling her pain without
making her "foggy."*

*When we finished, she sat up and slowly repeated all
we had said, with special emphasis on: "I can have the
medication when I request it?" We reassured her she had
understood us correctly. She leaned back in bed and
said in a low voice: "It might work, it seems plausible."
We suggested she might want to keep a log to record the
times she received the medication; the kind she received;
if the drug for pain relief was effective, minimally effective, or ineffective; length of time it took to attain pain
relief, and how long the drug(s) kept her comfortable.
She indicated she would like to keep account of how
she felt in a steno notebook. We told her we planned to
use her comments in conjunction with the nursing notes
to assist in titrating the correct amount of drugs she'd
receive. (A comparison of objective observations by
nursing staff combined with subjective comments by the
patient could be enlightening and useful data now and
in the future for this patient as well as others.)*

*Mrs. Ross asked a few questions about the drugs
ordered for her, that is, potency, side effects, and how
one drug compared to the other as to dosages ordered.
Demerol, she wished to avoid, if at all possible, for this
caused her to become "foggy" mentally. Dilaudid, she
decided not to use at this time, merely stating: "Let's
hold that in abeyance right now." (Although I did not
seek validation from her I wondered if use of this
powerful narcotic would mean to her that she was much*

sicker. Right then her need to deny any exacerbation of illness was paramount, if she was to make it to Texas.)

Mrs. Ross began the new regimen immediately by selecting Percodan. She related that this drug had controlled her pain fairly well in the past and did not have the effect of making her "foggy."

The first day, beginning at 1:40 PM, Mrs. Ross requested two Percodan tablets, and again at 5 and 9 PM. She took Seconal, 100 mg at midnight for sleep. Her notes, and those of the nursing staff, revealed that she was fairly comfortable after the second dose of Percodan. She recorded forty minutes as the time required to obtain a fair amount of pain relief. The following day she had the same drug and dosage at 1:45 AM, 9 AM, and 3:45 PM, with notes stating that pain relief was obtained in approximately thirty minutes. Pain was better controlled on the second day, she felt, with only a residual dull pain over her abdomen. Nursing notes revealed that Mrs. Ross appeared more alert and relaxed. She indicated her pleasure and relief at never waiting long for the nurses to bring her medication. It appeared that she was beginning to trust that the nurses would bring her medication without delay. The third day, she requested and received Percodan at 2 AM, 2 PM, and 11:30 PM. The latter dose she decided to combine with 100 mg of Seconal. She awakened the following morning and stated she had no pain! When I visited her several hours later, she looked serene and peaceful. She delighted in sharing the news with all the staff members. For the remainder of her hospital stay, twelve more days, she continued on the above regimen of two tablets of percodan every ten to twelve hours, combining her last dose, before sleeping, with 100 mg of Seconal. She was discharged to visit her relatives in Texas, taking with her the same medications for control of pain. (Note: Mrs. Ross lived for fourteen more days, eleven of which were spent with her daughter, Sandy, before requiring further hospitalization. Letters nursing staff received from both daughters after the funeral indicated that Mrs. Ross had indeed been able to complete her "unfinished business.")

It indeed seems strange that such a system of individualizing patient's pain medication does not occur to us more frequently. There's a strong tendency to become stereotyped in adhering to and perpetuating 3- to 4-hour pain orders when we know that pain differs widely in quality and quantity for each individual. How much more useful to have the patient involved in decision making based on information he gives to guide us in titrating the degree, duration, and efficacy of medication needed to forestall the onslaught of pain.

A crucial point, I believe, is to stay "on top of the pain," that is, prevent it from ever occurring. This kind of pain control relieves the patient from becoming dependent upon clocks and persons administering the drug. It permits him to complete his "unfinished business" without being consumed by pain, or to engage in those pursuits which make his remaining time both satisfying, meaningful, and serene, without the threat of pain.

The control and relief of pain should include the patient. As an active participant—receiver in the titration of pain control, the terminally ill patient knows his request for medication will be acted upon promptly, and that staff members are both interested and involved in the maintenance of pain relief.

He also knows that careful attention and respect will be given to his comments regarding the degree of pain he encounters, and that dosages will be raised or lowered accordingly.

Listening to the patient is often therapeutic in itself—both physical and mental distress can be relieved by being expressed to someone else. One patient summed it up by saying: "In listening, he took part of my pain with him."

A phenomenon noticed while working with terminally ill patients is their frequently voiced need to be "clear and mentally alert." They often elect, if given a choice, to stand moderate and even severe amounts of pain in order to maintain clarity of thought and speech. Pain at that particular time appears to be relegated to a lesser position in the need hierarchy. However, if anti-pain drugs are personalized to relieve the patient's discomfort, yet do not cloud his consciousness, much unnecessary suffering can effectively be avoided. If for some patients this is not possible, nursing personnel by monitoring the patient's reactions to discomfort can be responsive *to such variables by rendering anti-pain drugs when the need for alertness and conversation with significant others is less acute.*

Although only one experience has been related in personalizing the management of pain for the terminally ill patient, it appears possible to extrapolate the process in personalizing the management of pain for other terminally ill patients.

Personalized care should be the goal for all who are ill, particularly for those in pain. For those who are terminally ill and in pain personalized care must be the norm. Can we be content to settle for less?

Comments

Nurses and physicians obviously used their creative abilities in caring for Mrs. Ross. Although they at first adhered to the usual routine for controlling pain by administering medication every 3 to 4 hours, they eventually moved to another, more innovative and effective way of relieving her pain.

The client was able to participate in her plan of care, was able to make her own decisions, and not only benefitted personally but provided valuable data for personnel who would be able to use this experience to help other clients in similar difficulties. Encouraging independence and providing means by which she could plan her medication regimen to prevent pain made the client more comfortable and was a satisfying experience for personnel who could see the client's physical relief despite the fact that she was being given a reduced amount of medication.

Listening to the client and paying careful attention to her reports on the effects of her medication gave the client a sense of security and firmly reassured her that the personnel involved with her care were interested in her as a person.

This report is a good illustration of the successful way in which health team members can include the client as an active participant in assessing, planning, implementing, and evaluating his care; communication and cooperation are apparent, mutual trust and respect are integral parts of the activity, and the end result is quality care and satisfaction both for the client and for personnel.

SITUATION: MR. ADAM ZAPPELLE IN AN INTENSIVE CARE UNIT

Mr. Zappelle was 65 years old; he really looked younger, despite the ominous appearance of the ventilator at his side, which was making strange noises. The tube that protruded from the newly formed tracheostomy was surely frightening to him, also. The nurse who was just arriving for assignment to the intensive care unit looked briefly at Mr. Zappelle, rapidly assessed those needs that would demand first priority, then went to see what additional information she could obtain about him. She received some data about frequency of medications and the observations to make, but received little data about him as a person. No family members had been seen; no one was available who had personal knowledge about Mr. Zappelle. The record developed by the medical staff suggested he was being treated for an advanced carcinoma of the pharynx, and metastases had been detected in the lymph nodes of the neck. Primary symptoms were pain and an inability to eat because of a poor appetite. The nurse saw an anxious, frightened man with tense, taut muscles. In addition to the up-and-down motion and the sound of the ventilator bellows, sounds of the cardiac monitor added to the usual bustle of activity in such a unit. To provide further discomfort for Mr. Zappelle, a Foley catheter was in place, an intravenous infusion was running, and his arm was stabilized to an armboard to prevent him from moving it. These areas of assessment were apparent; no one could miss these in any review of client needs. The astute nurse had just arrived to care for the acutely ill persons on this unit and saw beyond Mr. Zappelle's obvious problems. As she spoke to him and introduced herself, he looked at her with eyes that seemed to reveal many messages. The nurse could not read all of the unvoiced messages, but she inferred he needed some comfort, some respect of himself as a person, some relief from many physical restrictions, some ease in breathing, and some understanding of what he was enduring.

The nurse decided that one of his major needs, at this point, was to communicate; his vital signs were stabilized sufficiently, the ventilator was helping his breathing problem, but his fear was still very obvious. Perhaps if he could communicate with someone and share his fears, the nurse and others on the medical and nursing teams could plan to cope with his problems. The nurse decided to suggest to him that he use a pencil and paper to tell her what he wanted and the things he wanted to say, because he could not express himself verbally. He was informed that the nurse would spend 10 to 15 minutes out of every 2 hours just talking with him, discussing the equipment around him, explaining its purposes and helping him to understand the medical therapy being planned for him.

Surely it was not the nurse's imagination, but Mr. Zappelle seemed to relax a bit after being told the nurse would visit him regularly. The visits with the nurse were profitable and revealing. She confirmed her suspicions that Mr. Zappelle was accustomed to being very independent. Obviously, being confined to bed in an intensive care unit was not conducive to independence. The next challenge to the nurse was to determine the activities in which he could become involved to assume some of his own care. Gradually he learned to care for the Foley catheter, learned to suction the mucus from his mouth, and became more able to turn himself at regular intervals as the intravenous infusions were reduced and finally eliminated. Encouraged by his increasing ability to care for himself his appetite for food returned; he began to eat better, selected foods he liked and preferred, and generally took on the glow of successful recovery. Although his progress to complete recovery would be prolonged, it was in a positive direction, promising to all but especially to Mr. Zappelle..

Comment

Assessment of obvious problems as well as subtle or covert needs is important in all care. Many of both types of problems were present in this situation and an astute nurse observed some discrete behaviors. The challenge of communicating with one who cannot speak was solved by planning new and different approaches to communication, and by implementing them. The client's obvious progression to a unit that was not an acute care area undoubtedly suggests that the approaches used by those caring for Mr. Zappelle were successful. The fact that he progressed to a point where he could assume increased responsibility for his own care also illustrates the effectiveness of these approaches.

The nurse was sensitive to the fact that Mr. Zappelle had lost his ability to communicate verbally; coping with such a handicap, whether it is temporary or permanent, necessitates a totally new body image construct. By carefully assessing the client's condition, the nurse can determine action that can be supportive to him.

SITUATION: SALLY SILLICK IN AN ADOLESCENT UNIT OF A GENERAL HOSPITAL

The adolescent years can be a serious time of life for a 15-year-old; it can be quite complicated when this growing-up phase includes coping with possible rheumatic fever.

When Sally Sillick was admitted to the adolescent unit of a general hospital, she complained of a very red, swollen, hot-to-touch, and painful left knee. Extensive examinations and tests established the diagnosis; careful observation for possible symptoms of carditis was done conscientiously. Immediate therapy included strict bed rest and a course of salicylates. Within 24 hours, the tenderness and swelling in her knee had subsided, but all other evidence confirmed the diagnosis of rheumatic fever. Treatment was to be prolonged and trying for this young girl, and her reaction to the diagnosis and proposed treatment was to withdraw.

Sally's mother was very attentive; she came to the hospital each day and spent many hours talking with Sally, reading to her, and exerting every effort to find something to stimulate her interest. Although her mother chatted with other young girls in the four-bed room, Sally showed no interest in joining any of the conversations. In fact, when the others tried to get her to socialize, she crawled deeper under the covers,

*making it clear to her peers and to her mother that she
would not socialize with them. Watching television was
her only interest; she would not read fiction, let alone
any of her school texts. Soon, there was evidence that
she was not eating, although she did agree to take medications brought to her, and permitted nursing personnel
to check her vital signs and involve her in the necessary
activities of personal hygiene. The nurse who was responsible for Sally's care was quite concerned, however,
and she could not think of any approach different from
that which she had already used to try to get through to
Sally and overcome her obvious withdrawal behavior.*

*To try to find a different approach to Sally, the
nurse assigned to her care asked that the next conference be devoted to Sally's problems as well as those
confronting the nurse who was trying to provide her
care. A discussion of Sally's behavior led to the suggestion that she may be experiencing some deeper anxiety that she had not yet expressed verbally. The diagnoses of withdrawal, refusal to eat, unwillingness to socialize, and lack of motivation were not difficult to define, but it was difficult to assess the underlying cause
of these diagnoses. The group members suggested that
the nurse who cared for Sally should pursue different
topics of conversation than she had used in the past to
find one that would evoke some reaction from Sally.*

*Armed with some new ideas from her group con-
ference, the nurse mentally preplanned various topics
she would introduce to Sally, and several of the subjects
had to do with girls' hobbies. A slight spark of interest
was kindled when the nurse mentioned knitting. She
pursued this topic cautiously, trying, in a judicious manner, to restrain her joy, hoping that the slight interest
she had evoked might be broadened into a healthy one.*

*Returning to the conference room that afternoon,
the nurse assigned to Sally's care gave a hopeful report,
and the group, now acting as consultants to the nurse,
provided her with another idea to suggest to Sally. One
of the children in the pediatric unit on the next floor
was anxious to have one of the new knitted sweaters
that so many of the children were wearing, but the
child's mother could not afford to buy her one. Would
it be possible to ask the child's mother to buy some
yarn and, at the strategic time, ask Sally to knit a
sweater for the little child? When the nurse followed
through with this suggestion, Sally brightened and*

*showed obvious enthusiasm for the first time since she
was hospitalized. The nurses were pleased, and Sally's
mother was happy and grateful for the apparent progress in Sally's attitude toward her illness and her required restrictions.*

*Unfortunately, Sally's enthusiasm for knitting was
short-lived. Just about a week after plans had been made
for her to knit the sweater, the nurse came into the
room after the physicians had been in to visit and found
Sally lying very quietly in bed, staring out the window.
A cheerful greeting from the nurse brought no response,
and it was apparent that she had lapsed into the same
type of withdrawal she had experienced previously. The
nurse attempted to talk about knitting the sweater, but
Sally did not respond. Abruptly, the nurse said: "Sally,
are you afraid?" Sally burst into tears, and in the next
hour, amid tears and sobs, she told the nurse how frightened she was of the "heart condition" she had, and how
she knew she would never be able to do what other girls
her age could do. The nurse was surprised to learn that
this was Sally's perception of her illness, when in fact,
her prognosis for complete recovery, with no residual,
was very good.*

*As soon as the nurse was able to do so, she called
the attending physician and discussed the events of the
day with him. He promptly called Sally's mother to
discuss the incident with her and to correct any misinformation she had about the illness. When the physician
came to see Sally and talked with her about what she
could expect and how hopeful she could be, Sally became an entirely different person. She became more
cheerful, had a healthier appetite, and became more
interested in her environment and in those around her.*

Comment

It can be assumed that Sally experienced an uneventful recovery after it was discovered she had been misinformed
about her illness and the misinformation was corrected. The
astute observations of the nurse in assessing withdrawal
symptoms and her willingness to discuss and consult with her
peers to get ideas and suggestions are all positive aspects of
the nursing process. The nurse continued to evaluate each of

the approaches she used to find a better or different way to provide for Sally's needs; she was keenly aware of Sally's varying moods and her reactions to the techniques used to provide the necessary care. Collaboration with the attending physician reinforced the nurse's role in sharing information with related health care workers; the physician's prompt response suggests he appreciated the nurse's alertness to the propitious moment to ask pertinent questions abruptly. Different phases of the nursing process and the different roles assumed by health care personnel on the health team can be identified in this situation.

SITUATION: MR. SEEHEW
IN AN INTENSIVE CARE UNIT

Mr. I. Seehew was 52 years old when he underwent surgery for the repair of a dissecting aneurysm. He was admitted to the intensive care unit as a critically ill person whose life-sustaining equipment included a respirator, an endotracheal tube, chest tubes, urinary bladder catheter, and intravenous equipment. He had experienced gastric bleeding and convulsions, and by the second week, postoperatively, he had not yet regained consciousness. Even though the life-sustaining equipment was removed, his vital signs remained stable.

Because he was in the unit for an extended period of time, the nursing staff was becoming "insensitive" to Mr. Seehew's needs and the nurses' reaction to him was becoming negative. His prognosis was apparently negative and the nurses who were tuned to caring for more acutely ill persons were rebelling at the idea of caring for this person who was stabilized although still acutely ill, and who did not require the kind of care nurses were accustomed to give in the "intensive, insensitive, expensive" unit. That the nurses rejected the client was apparent. Mrs. Seehew was his only relative and she became aware of the staff's feelings toward her husband. The nursing supervisor was informed about the situation by concerned nursing and medical staff members, and a meeting of the nurses was called to discuss the situation.

Through discussion, skillfully guided by the supervisor, the nurses' feelings about the client were revealed and explored. The revelation was not too surprising, and the nursing staff members should have been sensitive to what was going on before the meeting was called. However, it is sometimes necessary for a chain of events to occur before anyone becomes fully aware of what is happening in such a situation. The usual goal in the intensive care unit is to care for the client's immediate physiologic needs; nurses in the unit are especially skilled in the technical care of the critically ill. Because Mr. Seehew had remained in the unit for a longer period of time than is usual for most patients, most of the care for his physiologic needs was fairly well routinized. Having met these needs, the nurses should have proceeded to fulfill his other needs, but failed to recognize them. They were not consciously aware that their own behavior was contributing to Mr. Seehew's inadequate care. Also, the nurses had overlooked the needs of the client's wife who was going through a period of stress and crisis. Caring for and being aware of her psychologic needs were just as important as meeting Mr. Seehew's needs.

At the end of the group discussion, a number of questions were raised and the nurses tried to answer their own inquiries. As a result of their self examination, the following set of objectives was defined:

1. Discuss Mr. Seehew's plan of care with the medical staff to get information about the medical plan and to share the goals of the nursing plan,
2. Identify his level of physiologic needs and establish other needs the nurses can help to meet,
3. Establish a plan of caring for the client's wife and help her to meet her needs in a way similar to the plan being established for Mr. Seehew.

The nurses set these as the immediate, short-range goals; they knew that other long-range goals would soon be necessary, but immediate goals were the most important now, for the benefit of the client and to motivate and stimulate the interest of the staff nurses.

Each nurse on the staff of the unit felt deeply committed to accomplish the goals that had been established by the nursing group for the benefit of Mr. Seehew. Each nurse supported the other in her efforts to achieve the established goals. Communication between the medical staff and the nursing staff improved; each seemed to compete with the other to achieve the best performance *in taking care of Mr. Seehew. His wife responded positively to the increased concern demonstrated by the nurses; the staff's pleasure grew as they saw the success of their efforts.*

Within seven days from the time of the conference, Mr. Seehew was transferred to another unit in the hospital; a complete report of all his needs and the nursing care plan that was so successful while he was in the intensive care unit was shared with nurses who would now be caring for him. One month after he was transferred from the intensive care unit, Mr. Seehew regained consciousness. Sometime later, he was able to walk in his room and to function independently. His recovery was attributed to the success of the staff in assessing his and their needs, to their cooperative planning, to implementing a plan that was shared cooperately between medicine and nursing and later with other disciplines on the health team, as well as to the constant reassessment of established goals.

Comment

The success of the endeavor illustrated above depends largely on the honesty of the nursing staff with each other and the degree to which they have established mutual trust and respect. Willingness to reveal their true feelings about caring for a client usually is not spontaneous. When one has become caught in a routine that is obviously depersonalizing, conscious awareness of this error is not attractive to those involved. Nurses are to be commended when they use appropriate avenues to discuss what has happened to the process of client care when they realize it has or is threatening to deteriorate. Including the soul-searching self-assessment, as did these nurses in this situation, is commendable.

**SITUATION: MISS LOTT
IN A GENERAL HOSPITAL**

To carry out the nursing process with a client whose culture is different from that of the nurse presents quite a challenge. To better understand the behaviors of the client, Mona Lott, the nurse had to learn as much as possible about a different culture, to communicate in as many ways as possible with the client and her family, and to use all of her ingenuity and available resources to influence members of the nursing and hospital staff to go along with the suggested plan. The results were gratifying to the nurse and were appreciated by the recipients—the client and her family.

Some of the nurse's observations on Mona were direct; others were indirect. But, all observations contributed to increasing her knowledge about what illness means to the Navajo. Essentially, illness means that something is out of harmony—out of tune with nature. The Navajo believes that only the medicine man can cure illness; the white man's doctor can treat only symptoms. The medicine man tries to remove the evil that has caused the illness; the white man cannot do this. Mona was convinced that as soon as some of her symptoms were treated at the hospital, she would be allowed to return to her home where a ritual could be performed to make her well.

An assessment of her status convinced the nurse that Mona was losing her hope of getting well; she was beginning to despair of experiencing the ritual which would make her well.

Goals were directed to encourage hope; to accomplish this, another objective was necessary: some arrangements had to be made for the ritual. A major hurdle was to convince the hospital administrators that this ritual was necessary for the welfare and eventual recovery of the client. The hurdles proved to be surmountable, and arrangements were made to have the ritual performed in the hospital room.

To all who observed the abbreviated form of the ritual it was a tremendous experience. The actual rite was shorter than usual because it was performed in the hospital. Essentials of the rite were included, however, and we could see that efforts to arrange for the ritual were successful. It was not long before Mona began to respond to the treatment of the white man's doctor. Because she believed the evil that had caused her illness was removed by the medicine man's ritual, she now had a more positive outlook toward recovery. With renewed hope, Mona responded to medications so

promptly her recovery was phenomenal. The nurses had as-
sessed the primary problem Mona was experiencing and were
able to plan and implement methods to cope successfully
with the diagnosed problem. From the data gathered through
observation, it was concluded that the efforts were suc-
cessful. Knowledge, decisions, judgment, and collaboration
with members of the health team and the client's family were
all directed toward the desirable outcome for the client.

Comment

This example shows the importance of coping with that problem most important to the client. All of the treatment and
medications the client had received were of no benefit so
long as she believed the source of her illness, or evil, was still
present in her body. By providing the only person she believed could remove the evil, the health team was able to
provide treatment that helped her to recover; the client's
psychologic and physical states were responsive because she
was receptive. This report also illustrates the major role culture plays in working with and caring for people. Each person
responds as a total unit to others in his environment; the
physical, psychosocial, and cultural components of an individual blend harmoniously into one.

SITUATION: MRS. RUSSE
IN A GENERAL HOSPITAL

Mrs. Vi Russe was hospitalized for several weeks. Her
problem was chronic herpes zoster, and medication was
not controlling the pain. Mrs. Russe was taught to ad-
minister her own medication; her husband was involved
in the instruction sessions, and both seemed anxious to
have Vi at home again. Despite the apparent success of
all treatments, Vi's condition did not progress as it
should have or as it was expected to.
To determine the reason for stabilization in less than
a positive state, records were scoured for clues; confer-
ences were held with various health team members; and
discussions were conducted with Mrs. Russe and her

husband. Finally, when all data were assembled and analyzed, it was found that Mrs. Russe had regressed from a relative independent state to one of dependence; however, no real cause for the regression could be determined.

Conferences were held by the nursing staff members; the goal was to try to ascertain why the client's need for help in providing for her daily needs had increased and why her ambulation and socialization had decreased. To obtain some answers to these questions, the same nurse was assigned to her care as frequently as possible. The plan included frequent visits, a positive, friendly manner, and communication by word and action that people were interested in her; nurses were to be alert for any clues that might present themselves, and they were to encourage independence. Despite deliberate planning to meet these goals, only minimal results were achieved.

Evaluation and replanning led to a new approach. Less emphasis would be placed on independence; her state of dependence would be accepted; discussion of such matters as the dangers of prolonged bedrest would be limited; all these would be pursued while trying to anticipate and provide for as many of Mrs. Russe's needs as could be determined. After several days in which this latter approach was used, an evaluation conference revealed that Mrs. Russe was responding well to this indirect approach. She appeared to be taking more interest in her own care and expressed some desire to get out of bed more often. On several occasions she responded to conversation initiated by the other client in the room; this was something she had not done before. Gradually, she responded to treatment sufficiently to be discharged. She was still dependent on others for some assistance, but there was some movement toward increasing independence. The medical and nursing staff members concluded that Mrs. Russe was now sufficiently motivated to continue her positive progress. Follow-up visits at her home are needed to confirm this conclusion.

Comment

Though not presented in complete detail in terms of medications, treatment, or all of the problems with which Mrs.

Russe had to cope, this report suggests that the approach to planning and implementing any plan of care should be thoroughly individualized. The approach that was used for one client may not be effective for another. Some clients resent, whereas others respond well to, a direct approach. It is important for the nurse to read clues as well as she can and to make decisions and judgments based on her knowledge of human behavior to determine the approach she should use in any one situation.

SITUATION: MR. ZDROAK IN A GENERAL HOSPITAL

Mr. Zdroak had a cerebral vascular accident on Thursday. By Saturday morning his semicomatose state cleared. When the nurse entered his room he was sobbing; his left arm and leg were limp and motionless at his side.

The nursing process was triggered by the nurse's perception of the client's behavior; she assessed the client's state as discomfort and depression. She inferred that he was frustrated, frightened, and helpless to cope with his situation. The nurse's goal is to share with him her perception of his state, determine whether her perceptions are correct, and explore what this experience means to him. To initiate the conversation, the nurse said: "I know you are concerned about being unable to move your arm and your leg." The client replied: "Yes, I am very upset about it. My brother had the same thing happen to him some 5 years ago and he was helpless for 2 years before he died. I thought it just could not happen to me, but it has happened. I just don't want to become as helpless as my brother."

This response from Mr. Zdroak validated the nurse's perception, but she also found the reason for his concern—he had seen his brother in a similar state. The nurse, by her presence, by her well-phrased questions, by permitting appropriate pauses and silences during the conversation, is communicating to Mr. Zdroak that she is interested in him as a person, is concerned about his fears, and is willing and available to help him during the recovery process. Although some of the communication is nonverbal, the client responds positively to the nurse's approach. She is formulating judgments and making decisions while she is communicating with him and identifying his most immediate need—help in coping with his frustration and despair so that a rehabilitation program can be implemented. Gradually, the client began to accept the nurse, saw that she was willing to help him, and a beginning trust was established, which would grow and develop over a period of time.

The short-range goal was to begin a program of therapy for the client's paralyzed arm and leg. The nurse shared with him the plan of exercise and activity advised for him. He reacted by comparing the exercise program to one he had used on his farm: "We only exercise the animals legs after they are injured, if we think they will be able to use them again." No doubt Mr. Zdroak thought: "Maybe I'll be able to walk again." After thinking for awhile about the idea of exercise, the client stroked his left hand and arm and said: "There is no feeling, but they are warm; they are alive; maybe those exercises will help. I'll move my good arm and leg, and if you will help me move the other arm and leg, maybe I can do something besides stay in this bed, lying flat on my back." The communication from Mr. Zdroak told the nurse that he was receptive to exercise; he even suggested a way to implement the exercise plan.

The nurse eagerly picked up the cue the client provided, and gave him necessary instructions about how to exercise and how long to continue his effort so that he would not overtire himself.

Throughout the entire effort, the nurse encouraged the client to perform the exercise program and she continually evaluated his response to the activity. She continued to listen to him to pick up any cues that would suggest further acceptance of his true state, or to indicate any regression in attitude or physical state.

Mr. Zdroak's behavior throughout the exercise program validated the nurse's assumption that he associated exercise with recovery. His behavior told the staff members that he was no longer preoccupied with fear and pessimism but saw himself as increasingly capable of handling the demands of his situation, because he had been given the necessary help when he was physically unable to help himself.

Comment

The importance of accurate assessment cannot be over-emphasized. Careful and astute observation of crucial parameters is essential. It is also important for the nurse to validate her observations with the client. Does the nurse view symptoms and behavior only from her own perspective, or does she seek ways to communicate with the client to confirm the accuracy of her assessment? Having established the problem areas that are of major concern to the client, the nurse uses the cues he provides to develop a plan of care that will help him to cope with the problems identified. Because the goals of care were established by the mutual efforts of nurse and client, the evaluation phase of the process can proceed in an orderly systematic manner.

SITUATION: MR. ELDER IN A NURSING HOME

Mr. Elder was about 90 years old; he had muscle con-tractures of the knees, hips, elbows, shoulders, as well as extensive decubiti of the sacrum and lateral thigh. He had difficulty swallowing food, and was becoming mal-nourished because no one spent enough time to feed him. They did not have the time to wait until he coped with dysphagia sufficiently to get some food into his stomach. When a new nurse was transferred to the area where Mr. Elder was located, he was one of the first clients for whom a conference was scheduled. His mul-tiple problems made it obvious that Mr. Elder needed some very special care. The nurses discussed the prob-able cause of the decubiti and concluded that: he was turned from side-to-side infrequently, hence prolonged periods of lying in one position could easily cause decu-biti to develop; a malnourished state fostered skin ul-cerations and abrasions in multiple areas of his body. Problems experienced by Mr. Elder were identified as:
1. Decubiti needed immediate attention and care
2. Dietary intake was poor in quantity and quality
3. Mr. Elder was hard of hearing
4. There was no apparent means of sensory stimulation

5. *Attitude of staff nurses was "why worry about bed-sores when he is so sick he probably cannot live too long anyhow"*
6. *Because of the multiple care needs, more than one person should be assigned to care for him*

Having identified these as major problem areas, another session was held to determine the best way to cope with them.

Planning was done chiefly by the professional nurse at first, but her secondary aim was to motivate other nursing personnel to see Mr. Elder in a more positive way, to see his potential for relative recovery, and to implement measures of care, using their own initiative.

A 20-minute turning schedule was set, with two team members assigned to turn Mr. Elder at scheduled times. His right and left sides and abdomen were used in turning him, and he was never placed on his back because the decubiti on the sacrum were severe. Each time he was turned, the decubiti were washed, dried, and ointment was applied. A heat lamp was used regularly to promote drying and the tissue was treated very cautiously. These measures gradually were successful. Feeding was planned at short intervals, using small amounts of food with a high protein content, such as custards, soft cooked eggs, eggnog, and a special protein feeding.

A discussion of nurses' attitudes about caring for older people and the importance of taking care of the "living" rather than the "dying" person eventually made an impact on personnel. After a deliberate and continued instruction session with nursing aides, they began to spend more time with Mr. Elder, took the necessary time to feed him, turn him, and, eventually, to be patient enough to speak slowly and distinctly so that shouting at the hard-of-hearing Mr. Elder was no longer necessary. Communication was finally effective. After seven days of discussion and prodding by the head nurse, the decubiti were dry and granulation tissue had begun to appear around the edges of the ulcerated area. Mr. Elder began to respond by speaking to those around him more often. His increased dietary intake was beginning to show effects: he had more energy, became more alert, and was making more demands for attention. These evidences of progress stimulated the staff; they could see the results of their efforts and began to work harder to try to accomplish more. It was now a challenge to them to see who could do the most for Mr.

Elder. There was still a long way to go to full recovery, but the first steps had been taken.

Comment

Introducing a new face and some fresh ideas into a fairly stabilized situation can be a threat to personnel or it can produce qualitative results.

The newly assigned nurse described in this situation was a person-oriented practitioner who recognized the dignity of Mr. Elder and who visualized the constructive efforts that could be made on his behalf. Having the courage to lead personnel who had fallen into a routine of care in a different direction is not easy. It is essential and important, however, when the client's welfare is the ultimate goal. Using instrumental as well as expressive roles, this nurse effectively directed the staff toward assessing Mr. Elder's problems carefully, and to use initiative and originality in planning and implementing the care he required. Evaluation in terms of improved physical status is quite apparent; more subtle areas of providing sensory stimulation, for example, require more discreet measures.

SITUATION: MRS. FIDA IN THE HOSPITAL AND AT HOME

Mrs. B.I. Fida is a 28-year-old multipara. She had come to the hospital entrance, obviously in active labor, although her expected date of delivery was 4 weeks off. Diagnostic examinations had previously confirmed twins. Despite premature labor, she progressed normally through the different stages, and 8 hours after she was admitted to the labor room, she delivered twin boys. One boy, Twin A., weighed just less than 4 pounds and was normal in appearance. The other boy, Twin B., weighed just over 4 pounds and appeared to have possible mild hydrocephalus.

A spontaneous cry from each boy at birth brought the usual smile of joy to personnel in the delivery room. As could be expected, it was not very long before the mother asked anxiously: "Are they all right?" A very brief delay was evident before Mrs. Fida's question was answered. The doctor moved to her side after he completed a cursory examination of the infants, and with deep and sincere compassion, couched his words into the type of phrases that would tell the mother she had borne twin boys; one appeared quite normal, but the other appeared to have mild hydrocephalus. Mrs. Fida had a great deal of confidence in her physician, and her trust in his truthfulness was apparent; she cried and was obviously distressed at the information she had received, but she seemed to cling to the careful use of the word "mild" hydrocephalus. The doctor promised Mrs. Fida he would see her in a few hours, after she had time to recover from the effects of some of the medications. He promised to spend as much time as she wished, talking about the children. Though the mother's disappointment was still very obvious, she appeared satisfied with the doctor's explanation and his promise to come back to discuss the babies' welfare very soon.

When the doctor left the delivery room, Mrs. Fida asked the nurse if she could see the babies. The incubators were moved close enough for her to see the infants, and the nurse raised Mrs. Fida's shoulders and head so she could look at the newborn boys. When she was no longer able to keep her shoulders and head raised from the table, Mrs. Fida laid her head back on the arms of the nurse and sobbed gently; the nurse stood silently, then gradually lowered Mrs. Fida's head as her sobs began to subside. Words were not important now, nor were they necessary at this stage. The mere presence of the nurse, holding Mrs. Fida's hand, and communicating by her facial expression and touch that she understood and sympathized, was all that was necessary at the moment.

The doctor stood at the delivery room door with Mr. Fida, and together the doctor and nurse told him the news and showed him the babies, as they had the mother. Mr. Fida, too, was tearful and disappointed. The doctor and nurse left the room at that time so that mother and father could be alone to share the grief and disappointment that always accompanies the birth of a less than normal child.

While the parents were grappling with their reactions to this event and trying to cope with their feelings, the nurse was having a similar problem. She felt it was necessary for her to acknowledge her own reactions to the birth of such a child, and to be aware of her feelings of disappointment, certainly different in caliber than those of the parents but, nevertheless, very real. Her immediate impulse was to retreat, to remove herself from the area, but this was a fleeting thought. Actually, she knew she would care for the mother, and deliberately began to plan the way to approach that care. She decided she would show interest in both children, she would provide every possible opportunity for mother and father to discuss their feelings about the twins with her, especially Twin B. who had hydrocephalus. Also, the nurse obtained as much information as she could that would be useful to the Fida family, and planned to make opportunities available for them to see other parents who had successfully coped with children who were born with similar handicaps. Above all, the nurse and the doctor were convinced of the importance of being honest with the parents, and the parents knew they could depend on the forthrightness of these two persons. Having established their trust and confidence in the physician and nurse, Mr. and Mrs. Fida had taken the first major step in the long road to adjusting to their new role, that of being the parents of a handicapped child.

As the normal twin progressed in his feedings, and his weight increased, Mrs. Fida became more encouraged; gradually the nurse involved Mrs. Fida in the feeding activity, and this was especially helpful in raising her morale. Initially, the infant feeding was somewhat difficult for the mother; apparently she would think more vividly, at each feeding, about the other twin who was not on the same feeding schedule. Before long, the nurse included the mother in Twin B.'s feeding schedule too, bringing her in to observe the infant feeding. As the mother became more assured of the baby's ability to take the feedings, she was more confident of her own abilities, and assisted with feeding both babies in a short time.

Both babies reached a fairly stable state, and Mrs. Fida had sufficiently recovered so that she was ready to be discharged from the hospital. Two children at home, one in the fourth grade at school and one in the first grade, concerned the parents; how would they react to the new baby who was "different?" The parents were encouraged to discuss with the children the fact that the new babies would be coming home later, and that one of the babies was different from most. The children were encouraged by the parents that they would be able to work together as a family to help the new babies, especially Twin B. The approach to these discussions was a positive one, stressing the valuable opportunity available to the family to care for such a special child.

Having coped with discussing the new babies with the children at home, the parents were faced with another challenge—the reactions of relatives and friends. When the parents verbally expressed their concerns about these reactions, the nurse encouraged them to continue their positive approach to the twins, and operate on the premise that their positive and matter-of-fact attitude and manner would become a role model for observant relatives and friends. Instructions to the parents were realistic; they were told that the course of events would not be totally smooth; there would be times the parents would be discouraged, there would be occasions when it would be most difficult to put up a positive front. To cope with such occasions, the nurse and doctor provided the parents with names, addresses, and phone numbers of some professional persons who would be available to them when they found it difficult to cope with the problem. They were also given the name of a parents' organization where they could meet others caring for exceptional children.

The Fida children were eagerly waiting for their mother to return home from the hospital; to the parents' relief, they did not seem worried that one of their brothers would be "different." (Such is the innocence of youth.) Between the day Mrs. Fida returned from the hospital and the day the twins were brought home, many hours were spent in talking with the children about their responsibilities when the new babies came home. The youngsters were equal to the task before them, and Mr. and Mrs. Fida began to settle slowly into a more comfortable role than they thought would be possible.

The first encounter with close relatives was not nearly so traumatic as the parents feared it would be—perhaps because they had succeeded so well in developing their own abilities to cope with the situation and in preparing the children for the new babies' arrival. Not *all days were smooth, and suggested resources were used on numerous occasions. However, all were coping with the situation and were making constructive efforts to support Mr. and Mrs. Fida in every possible way.*

Comments

The emotionally laden event of the birth of a handicapped child poses major challenges to personnel who care for the child and/or the parents involved. This situation illustrates how important it is for the nurse to be aware of her own feelings and reactions, essentially assessing her own needs and problem areas before she will be able to help the clients for whom she is responsible. Conscious, deliberate assessment and determining ways to cope with acknowledged assets and limitations are essential steps in the process of planning for the care of the client who needs some professional assistance.

The care process illustrated in this situation takes place in the hospital initially, but the nurse moved beyond the immediate situation to plan ways in which the client could cope with anticipated problems in the home setting. Forecasting and predicting are not essentials of nursing, but assuming and hypothesizing are innate qualities that contribute to the qualitative performance of the nurse. Astute listening to the client's fears and concerns as she prepares to go home from the hospital will provide the nurse with cues that can help her to plan with the client for anticipated eventualities. Follow-up visits by the nurse to the home, or return visits of the client to the hospital or clinic make data available from which the effectiveness of the planning in preparation for the return to the home can be determined.

SUMMARY

The situations cited in this chapter are far from inclusive for all types of encounters which could confront nurses. The goal of these reports is to suggest the variety of age groups, settings, and problem areas the client may present. It will be necessary to devise different methods of coping with client problems, depending on the variables identified in each encounter. The orderly thought processes suggested in the four phases of the nursing process, should make it easier for the nurse to cope with client problems.

chapter five

The Future of
the Nursing Process

In the preceding chapters, the development and application
of the nursing process supported the belief that this process is
vital, ongoing, goal-directed, and logical. Hence, it is not only
oriented to the present, but to the future. Its focus toward
the future implies a continuum, linking the present to the
future in a forward thrust.

The future of the nursing process cannot be predicted
without knowing the events, trends, and changes expected.
Speculations and predictions for mankind will have an impact
upon how, where, by whom, for whom, and when the
nursing process will be utilized.

It may be well to ponder expectations for man in the
future. Since the soaring sixties are part of history, recalling
the events of the past can give direction to planning for the
future. The idea of change is now an accepted part of life,
and it is safe to say that the only thing that can be predicted
with certainty is the fact that change will occur. The surge of
the seventies will present more change than that experienced
in the sixties.[1] "Change is the process by which the future
invades our lives."[2]

When discussing change, it is important to think in terms

of its rate and direction. For " . . . to define the content of change must include the consequences of pace itself . . . ."[2] A number of examples can illustrate the rate of change with which the human race must cope. One example is the economic growth rate of the United States. It took this country two centuries to reach the 1 trillion-dollar milestone in goods and services per year. It is expected to take less than 10 years to reach the 2 trillion milestone.*

Each person, whether professional or lay, can set up a unique list of what will be the major health problems of the seventies. At this early time in the decade, it seems clear that among the problems will be the following: (a) Pollution—air, water, land; contributing to this problem is that of overpopulation and the poor distribution of population. As more people occupy the earth, the amount of waste increases (liquid, solid, and gaseous). Crowding creates noise pollution, the metabolic processes of increasing numbers of people create more body waste and increased food consumption creates more garbage. Each of these contributes to mental and physical health problems. (b) Drugs—persons who take drugs, the care of persons who use drugs, and the reasons drugs are taken are of major concern. What makes a person, regardless of age, turn to drugs? Finding the answers to this question as well as coping with the problems created by drug users will be one of the major challenges of the seventies.

From an economic standpoint, coping with the rising cost of health care will be another of the major problems of the seventies. Many politicians, both those running for office as well as those already holding office, will focus on this problem. The debate about the involvement of the federal government, the never-ending questions about the extent to which the federal government should or should not be involved in financing health care, the way the state and federal governments should be responsible or share responsibility, and how they can do this without usurping the responsibility of local governments, are vital issues to be resolved during the seventies.

Continuing technical advancement without concomitant

*In numerals, 2 trillion looks like this: $2,000,000,000,000. To visualize 2 trillion dollars, a feat difficult for most of us, make 2,000 billion-dollar heaps.[2]

development, or the lagging development of the philosophic, ethical, and moral aspects of these advances are already presenting problems and may become greater problems in the future. The impact of these developments upon man and his environment, particularly those relating to genetic engineering or the question of designating the time of death, will be hard questions to be answered in the seventies; the term "sobering" may be far more accurate. The prevention of illness will be emphasized in the seventies as well as curative and rehabilitative aspects of medicine.

How do these relate to the nursing process? These will be among the issues pertinent to nursing and necessary to the nursing process. To illustrate: With emphasis on economics and on providing quality health care for the consumer of health services, a major issue will be the number of personnel needed, the kind of personnel, their training and education, their roles in health care, and their responsibilities. As more persons enter the area of nursing, can the consumer of nursing expect that more nurses will mean better care? Do nurses expect that the terms "more" and "better" can be equated?

The United States is a nation with some of the best medical resources known anywhere in the world. Yet, its infant mortality rate is greater than that of at least ten other advanced countries. In addition, in a nation where only 5% of the national income goes to 20% of its families at the lowest end of the economic ladder—where malnutrition is a major problem, where care and inoculations are unknown—rectifying these conditions is a challenge for the seventies.[1]

Toffler suggests that future shock "may well be the most important disease of tomorrow." He defines future shock as "... a time phenomenon, a product of the greatly accelerated rate of change in society .... It is culture shock in one's society." It is his belief that man handles technologic innovation by going through these phases—idea creation, idea application, and idea diffusion.[2] To paraphrase Toffler and apply the phases to nursing, use of the nursing process would involve three phases: (a) There must be a creative, feasible idea and the suggestion that here is a situation in which nursing can be of help; here is an area in which nursing offers

some expertise to resolve or prevent a problem from developing. (b) The process must have a practical application. Having
identified the area of need, assessed the problem or potential
problem areas, and arrived at a plan for coping, there must be
some action. This action includes implementing as well as
evaluating aspects of the process. Constant recycling through
phases is an inherent part of the process. (c) The third phase
in the utilization of the process involves "diffusion through
society." Translated into the language of nursing, this involves convincing those who do nursing that orderly movement through the process insures the "how" of nursing, it
insures the systematic and orderly movement through necessary phases of nursing so that problems of clients can be
thoroughly assessed, action for coping can be planned and
implemented, and a final and continual evaluation is as essential as is each of the other three phases of the process. Thus,
challenges for the future of society, of health care, and of
nursing care are coming into focus. The nursing process is the
significant process to meet some of these challenges.

The future of the nursing process is seen from four points
of view: (a) continuing development and refinement of the
process itself, (b) contribution toward the growth and development of the profession of nursing through its use, (c)
influences upon the personal and professional growth and
the development of users of the nursing process, and
(d) improvement of the health status of recipients of the process.

As nurse practitioners continue to use the nursing process
in a deliberate way, its components and component elements
are likely to be refined. Improved history taking, more accurate nursing diagnoses, more effective priority setting, improved design of nursing care plans, more astute specifica-
tions of expected client behaviors, more effective recording
of observations about the client, more sensible, purposeful
and effective nurse actions, more emphasis on evaluation as
well as on the development of tools of evaluation, better
judgment concerning what to communicate to whom, when
to communicate and how, are goals of the continuing
development of the nursing process.

Numerous authors have developed tools and technqiues which are incorporated into the nursing process. Continuing development, testing, and refinement of these tools in a variety of health care settings and with the nurse and other nursing and health team members are in order. Narrowing the lag that exists between the discovery of new knowledge, new methods, and their incorporation into nursing practice deserves a serious theoretic base to serve as the framework for the nursing process.

The contribution toward growth and development of the profession of nursing through the use of the nursing process is easily evidenced. Since the heart of nursing practice is the designation and solution of client problems, any theories or scientific materials developed to explain, direct, or influence nursing practice will contribute to the quality of service rendered the client and hence advance the profession and sanction its place as designated by society. A case in point would be the study and analysis of the content of nursing care plans. In Chapter 3, it was recommended that nursing care plans be developed in their entirety and retained for future study and analysis. Well-designed and complete nursing care plans would contribute a wealth of data about a client, his problems, solutions to those problems, and the effectiveness of these solutions. Research is inherent in the process. Hunches, observations, and speculations lend themselves to further research and testing. Nursing care plans can be analyzed according to many variables—age, sex, educational level, level of wellness, level of illness, common problems, unique problems, solutions and their effectiveness, the predictable level of success from alternative solutions, determining the status of solutions. The careful, analytic extraction and testing of data will more than likely contribute to the development of nursing theory. Nursing care plans, nursing histories, and associated observations and results can be used to develop model care plans for males and females of a particular age, with a particular problem, having certain resources and in a particular setting. These models can enhance the nurse's role as a client specialist.

When considering the influence of the nursing process

upon the nurse's personal and professional growth and development as a person and as a practitioner, a few topics need to be considered. For example: the nursing process as a process and functional entity should be a major component of continuing education, which would include its present use and reflect additional areas for use in a practice setting. The problem-solving that results from the nursing process is a fruitful area, replete with a multitude of situations that could be shared with colleagues for their enlightenment and reaction.

The nursing process lends itself to the nurse's own quest for self-improvement. Continuous evaluation of one's intellectual, interpersonal, and technical skills and one's perceptual, communicative, and decision-making ability will reveal strengths and limitations. Interest in enhancing one's strengths and minimizing one's limitations gives direction for study and the selection of programs, workshops, and professional associations and interactions. Improvement in areas of history-taking, nursing diagnoses, and listening, to mention a few, can be a lifelong endeavor. Increasing one's accuracy in problem-solving and in predicting the impact upon client behavior are important factors in experiencing success in nursing practice. The continuing focus on self-improvement results in the better use of self and improved contribution to citizens. In summary, the nursing process could be viewed as an effective method to prevent and minimize obsolescence.

For the citizen, the more knowledgeable, confident, creative, and person-centered the nurse is, the more likely the client will benefit. Whether his situation demands that wellness be maintained, care be given during acute or chronic illness or compassionate support rendered if he is dying, he will be the recipient of the best care the nurse has to offer. The nurse, too, will be stimulated to continue her self-development, as she reaps the feeling of accomplishment from giving her best. Inherent in this feeling of success is a realistic appraisal of oneself and the client situation. It involves being able to accept a setback without being unduly crushed, being able to strive forward despite odds, and being convinced that one's contribution is the best at a particular time.

The client further benefits by being an active participant

in the identification and resolution of his problems. It enhances his personhood, his need to remain a thinking, feeling person whether he is well or ill, and his need to maximize the well portion of his being even though he is afflicted by some disability.

The nursing process contributes to the nurse's feeling of camaraderie with other members of the health team. She places value on her contributions and enhances the success of herself and the health professionals by sharing her perceptions and goals for the client. She is, in turn, enhanced by being open and receptive to suggestions of nursing and health team members.

Inherent in each point of view relating to the future of the nursing process is the research process. Presently, the need for clinical research is generally recognized by nurse practitioners, and it is predictable that the quantity and quality of clinical nursing research will improve in the seventies. The need for increased research in nursing practice is documented in *Abstract for Action*, a report of the National Commission for the Study of Nursing and Nursing Education. The report clearly points to the need for a body of facts and a set of probabilities to guide or assess the nursing care of citizens. A clear knowledge of the differences in the benefits to the client from nursing interventions and establishing means to assess the results of varied interventions are based upon sound research.[3]

Research plays an important role in the development and refinement of the nursing process and in the development of nursing science. Sharing the results of research can benefit the nurse and client directly. The nursing process not only opens the way for research into a multitude of problems but each component with each of its elements is itself a fruitful area for research. Fox has developed a useful model for identifying research problems in nursing. The model is based upon the nursing process and includes numerous helpful suggestions for research by nurses alone or by nurses in collaboration with other health professionals. Summarizing the suggestions of Fox,[4] the following types of research studies may be undertaken: (a) those related to health needs, health personnel consulted about health needs, and the medical and nursing care plan; (b) those related to decisions inherent in the nursing process; (c) those related to the professional role and the legal limit of the practice of nursing; (d) those related to the setting in which the nursing process is utilized; (e) those related to the utilization of the nursing process by nurses with varying backgrounds in education and experience; (f) those related to the roles of the client, his family, and other professional and nonprofessional personnel in implementing the nursing care plan; (g) those relating to the impact of direct nursing care upon the client, and (h) those relating to the communication of data.[4]

Specifically, any of the following studies, as well as a multitude of others, could be undertaken with the hope that the results would contribute to the continuing development of the nursing process, comprise a nursing science, and contribute to an increase in the caliber of care rendered to citizens:

1. Comparative studies of nursing histories taken by nurses with differing educational and practice backgrounds and functioning in a variety of settings.
2. Studies of the utilization of the nursing history in the development of the nursing care plan.
3. Studies of the client's reaction to self-completion of the nursing history form, with and without personal interview.
4. Studies of the number and kind of decisions made based on data of the nursing history.
5. Comparative studies of the number and kinds of decisions made by nurses in varying settings and with different backgrounds of education and experience.
6. Studies of whether a selected number of nurses, given the same set of data, would make the same nursing diagnoses. If there is variation, studies of this variation according to education, experience, and culture of the nurses.
7. Studies of how different citizens with a similar health problem resolve this problem.
8. Studies of varying patterns of problem resolution ac-

cording to age, sex, geographic location, socioeconomic level, and educational and cultural background.

9. Studies to analyze the first encounter of the nurse and client in terms of why the client sought out the nurse. Studies to determine if the nurse was the first member of the health team to enter the client into the health care system or if the encounter resulted from his prior interaction with a physician or other health team member.

10. Studies to define the client's role in the development of the nursing care plan.

11. Studies to determine factors that comprise the rationale for setting priorities for client problems. A study of whether this priority setting is affected by differences in the nurse's education and experience and those of the client. Comparative studies of priority setting for client problems, as designated by the nurse and the client. If there is a conflict in priority setting, study the factors inherent in the conflict.

12. When eliciting solutions to client problems, studies should be done to determine how to recognize the best solution.

13. Studies of the rationale used by nurses in selecting a specific nursing action to resolve a problem.

14. Studies to determine factors inherent in the nurse's decision to refer or not refer a client problem to another health care professional or another agency.

15. Studies of perceptions and observations about the client that are recorded and shared in contrast to those withheld. Analytic studies of the data withheld and the rationale for withholding them. Studies of the nurse's education and experience in contrast to the quantity and quality of data withheld.

16. Studies to determine variations of and common solutions made by nurses in different settings when confronted with a given client problem, a designated number of staff, and selected equipment and supplies.

17. A study of the rationale for delegating actions to be performed by members of the nursing team rather than by the nurse herself.

18. Studies of the impact of agency policies on the number,

kinds, and quality of decisions made by the nurse relative to assessing, planning, implementing, and evaluating care.

19. Studies to develop tools to evaluate the impact of nurse actions on client behavior.
20. Studies to determine the client's role in evaluating the nursing care rendered to him.
21. Studies of the impact of the client's evaluation on subsequent nurse actions designated to solve problems.
22. Studies to determine the extent to which nurses transfer or reproduce decisions utilized in one situation to another.
23. Studies of inherent factors in a situation that foster or deter the transfer or reproduction of decisions.
24. Studies to determine why, when, what, and how nurses use research findings and incorporate them into their use of the nursing process.

In addition to recommended nursing research studies, it is imperative that nurses use the research findings related to human behavior and incorporate these into nursing practice.

Experiences in nursing have suggested two subject areas in particular that warrant exploration—periodicity and territoriality. The limited data already obtained from applications of these two concepts to nursing suggest there is a vast and rich potential that will contribute qualitatively to improved nursing and client care.

Periodicity is that cycle through which all living matter moves; the cycle is characterized by peaks and troughs in a regular pattern. Periodicity is also known as biologic rhythm, circadian rhythm, body rhythm, body clock, and a variety of other labels. The cyclic nature of the physical environment is discernable in the changing seasons of the year, in changing from day to night, in the blossoming of flowers and their return to seed, and in the annual harvesting of fields. The cyclic nature of the human body is evident by mood swings that people experience on a daily, monthly, or seasonal basis, by daily and monthly fluctuations in body weight, by the increase and decrease in appetite on a cyclic basis, by the sleep-wake cycle, and by many other parameters.

The advent of space travel has accelerated the need for understanding the timing adjustment of the body clocks. Intercontinental travel by jet planes provides speedy movement across date lines, yet it has become necessary to plan time schedules to allow body clocks to adjust to the change. For example: business men who travel to Paris must allow a 24- to 48-hour period for body systems to synchronize with the surrounding environment to provide for optimum functioning.

When one attempts to apply this concept of periodicity to client care, a number of questions are raised. To what extent is the client's body clock considered when planning for medication administration? Studies show that people are more susceptible to medication effects at certain times of the 24-hour period than at other times of the day. The peaks and troughs of metabolic activity account for this difference in receptivity to medication intake. Can nurses contribute to the collection of data that will provide a profile of client periodicity patterns? Are there certain times of the day when clients may be more mentally alert, more receptive to instructions about health care, about rehabilitation measures, about taking medications at home?

These are some of the many questions one can raise that relate to the concept of periodicity. Though time and study will be necessary to provide more complete data, the work should be initiated. Gradual but sure inroads into such concepts will be qualitatively beneficial to the client and to the nurse.

The concept of territoriality is associated with that area of space (earth, air, or water) a person defines and defends as his own. This is a relatively new concept in the natural and behavioral sciences. Studies show, however, that animate beings possess an inner compulsion to own their own territory and they exert a marked effort to defend it. Some authors see the territorial nature of man as a genetic trait that cannot be eradicated.[5] If one accepts this inherent quality in man, a number of questions can be raised relative to the territorial rights of clients with whom nurses function.

How does the client's territory concern the nurse? When

a nurse enters a client's home, it is not difficult to identify territorial rights and respect them. When a client comes to a clinic, a hospital, or other agency to seek help from health personnel, his territory grows smaller but does not vanish. It becomes a more circumscribed area of smaller dimensions, surrounding his person. In the hospital, the client's territory is usually limited to the area surrounding the bed, including the bedside table, the chair, and the bed itself. Clients usually refer to the lack of privacy in the hospital as a violation of personal space rather than an invasion of territory.[6] A certain amount of intrusion of personal space by personnel is necessary and expected when a person becomes ill. Being aware of the client's personal space is important to his care and the nurse must be concerned with his reaction to her intrusion. Responses to actions of others can change as one becomes ill. An event to which one would not react when healthy may create a marked reaction when ill. An intrusion or invasion of one's space or territory can represent a threat to the ill person. The reaction to the threat is essentially one in which the inherent drive to defend one's property is activated. The nurse must think of this mechanism when she is observing the client's behavior and assessing his situation.

A study by Crenshaw revealed 45 incidents in which 30 patients described what they perceived as unnecessary invasions of privacy. She assumed that invasion of privacy is one manifestation of the invasion of personal space. More than half of the invasions were by nursing personnel, most of whom were professional nurses.[7]

Though disciplines of anthropology, sociology, and psychology have studied this concept of space and territory, nursing has made only minor inroads into this subject. However, the fascinating potential of exploring this concept to determine its possible application to nursing should prove very exciting to practicing nurses. Those with pioneer spirits will find a great deal of data on which they can build some hunches, suggest some hypotheses, and explore realistically, in some depth, when helping clients in a variety of settings. Fertile areas for discovery can stimulate more growth and development in the nursing profession than has yet been realized. The major ingredients needed are a willing mind and enthusiasm for the continued improvement of self and service to others.

Thus, the nursing process can give rise to areas for nursing research, and the tools and data realized through the deliberate use of the nursing process can provide data for that research.

The quality of the nursing process in the practice of nursing and its involvement in research in nursing practice will be the basis for the certification of nurse specialists. This recognition for members of the profession by the membership will designate a high level of quality in service rendered to citizens. Among means to be utilized as evidence to support claims of excellence will be written descriptions of problem-solving or the use of the nursing process in a selection of nurse-client encounters. These descriptions will be subject to peer review. The evaluation inherent in the process itself, followed by an evaluation by peers incorporating standards of practice, supports the conviction that nurse practitioners have accepted the fact that they are accountable for these actions. While nursing has already agreed to accept this responsibility, citizen demand that health care personnel, political leaders, lawyers, and businessmen, to mention a few, be accountable for their actions will be increased and strengthened during the seventies.

Accountability suggests responsibility, an obligation to answer to someone. Legally, a nurse can be held accountable for her actions as well as her inactions.[8] Inherent within this obligation is the suggestion that the nurse is expected to have certain basic knowledge; she is obliged to make decisions, and to use judgment based on that knowledge. Within this context she is responsible for taking appropriate actions, whether dependent or independent.

Implementing independent actions by the nurse requires careful adherence to the nursing process to determine the scope of her responsibility and to insure qualitative fulfillment of actions necessary to help the client. As dependent actions are necessary, the nurse visualizes responsibilities along several avenues; she continually keeps in mind her responsibility to the client and his family, yet simultaneously is aware of her accountability to herself, to other nursing and health team members, and to her employer, if she is not an independent practitioner. Hence, this mosaic of accountability and responsibility takes on many dimensions. As these facets continually present themselves to the nurse practitioner, she is accountable for taking some action. If no action is taken when one is necessary, or when a legal action can prove a nursing action should have been taken, then the nurse is accountable. Thus, future responsibility is inherent in all present acts.

The primary focus for the nurse is the client and his problems. For helping the client to cope with actual or potential health needs, the nurse is directly accountable to him. Because the client is always viewed as an integral part of a family unit, the nurse is accountable to the client's family, in either a primary or a secondary way, or in a direct or indirect way.

Every nurse is accountable to herself. She knows best her intentions and she can best explain to what extent she is accountable. Usually, if the nurse is comfortably sure in her own mind that she has measured up to the demands of accountability to herself, then her accountability to others can be coped with successfully.

Accountability for solving the client's problems is shared by all members of nursing and health teams. There is vertical and horizontal accountability between and among team members. A liaison exists because of their mutual concern, the welfare of the client. Also a collaborative and an ethical role exists among personnel. The nurse is primarily responsible for instrumental functions of group cohesion as well as for the expressive functions of moving the group toward defined goals.

Another facet of accountability and responsibility is the willingness to share experiences through the professional publication of practical experiences. The nurse involved in using the nursing process will accumulate qualitative and quantitative physiologic and behavioral data about a client, which are available to few persons. The critical analysis of these data will render valuable information to serve as guidelines for the nurse's future actions. In addition to benefits to herself, the nurse has a professional responsibility to share these data with her colleagues, not only to enlighten them, but to stimulate their thinking and to propose ideas to a forum for reaction, refinement, and development by other members of the nursing profession. This sharing fosters the growth and development of the profession. The personal accumulation of valuable data benefits only one or two persons. Sharing this information with one's colleagues extends its value many fold. Not only will the value of the data be made known, but weaknesses and inaccuracies will be pointed out in an objective way, which, in turn, should benefit the sharer of that information. Solutions to problems, reactions of clients to solutions, the development of techniques and procedures, the recognition of problems unique and common to a person and/or setting, would serve as the basis for professional writing. Publishing the results of research by nurse practitioners gives the reader a basis for making judgments about the results and also gives her some knowledge of the research that has been completed, eliminating duplication. The published research study can serve as a model for future research.

Participating and writing in conjunction with other members of the health team can foster relationships and mutual understanding of each contributor's point of view and role. This health team and interdisciplinary collaboration is strategic in those settings and with those client problems that involve combined input from the nurse, the physician, the dentist, the pharmacist, the social worker, and so on.

In addition to its future role in research, the nursing process will play a significant part in fulfilling resolutions passed by the membership of the National League for Nursing and the American Nurses Association in 1971 and 1972,[9] respectively, and which have an impact on the future health care of citizens. Selectively, resolutions urge a speedy passage of health legislation which would afford high quality health care readily accessible to all segments of society. All aspects of health care services should be available, with greater emphasis on preventive as well as therapeutic aspects and with special attention to include financing mechanisms and appropriate cost control. It was resolved that a conference on health care be held to discuss the full range of preventive services, manpower needs, facilities, financing, and distribution of services. Emphasis on the use of home health services should be continued and action initiated and maintained to avoid duplication of such services at the community level. Existing home health care agencies presently providing client care should be used in any community level development, restructuring, or reorganization of health care services.

One resolution included a statement that skilled nursing is a composite of on-going observation, judgment, management, counseling, teaching, and direct care as well as the implementation of a nursing care plan in conjunction with medical orders. The nursing care plan must be evaluated and revised as indicated, and the client's needs and responses must be documented. Inherent in this resolution is national sanction for the nursing process. Another resolution stated that nursing shares responsibility for the health and welfare of the community and of the individual with health problems. A resolution was also passed, reaffirming preventive nursing care to the family as a unit and, in the event the client dies, support for the continuing services needed by the family.

Other resolutions reaffirm the commitment to care for clients with cancer, to improve the care and services to the elderly, and to participate actively with health care professionals and parents in planning and meeting the needs of mothers and children. Significantly, a resolution has been passed to exercise the *Code for Nurses* and to provide a mechanism for reporting and handling incompetent, unethical, or illegal practice. This resolution supports the emphasis placed upon the profession's accountability for its product or practice. The nursing process, with its built-in evaluation, would be the effective means for implementing this accountability.

It was resolved that peer review be provided in every health care facility to maintain standards of care. Inherent in this resolution is support for high-quality nursing practice for the citizen and the professional maturity which comes with the willingness to accept responsibility for one's acts and a desire to subject them to the scrutiny of one's peers. What better way is there to supply evidence that the nursing process has been used than nursing histories, nursing diagnoses, nursing orders, nursing care plans and their revisions and/or modifications? Another resolution stated that the Congress for Nursing and the divisions of practice develop mechanisms whereby clinical specialists define their role, qualifications, and responsibilities in nursing practice.

Learning programs in both the basic and continuing education programs were called upon to provide learning opportunities for competence in primary health care practice. The nursing process can be used effectively by the nurse engaged in primary health care. Continued education received considerable emphasis. The nursing process affords an almost endless number of topics and directions that can be pursued based on data obtained about clients, their problems, and solutions.

Many other resolutions were passed—all directly or indirectly geared to improve health services to the citizen. Some were related to supporting just remuneration for nursing services and prepaid health plans providing payment for nursing services. Others related to the need for effective health legislation. A nationwide moratorium on licensing additional health occupations was supported, as were sound licensing laws. The commitment to individual accountability and individual licensure as essential to high quality safe care was strongly reaffirmed. All resolutions will have an implication for the immediate and distant future. The nursing process as a process and its outcomes are strategic to fulfill these client-centered resolutions. ·

Results of the study of nursing and nursing education by the National Commission for the Study of Nursing and Nursing Education broadly outline the need to increase clinical nursing research and research related to nurse education. It confirms the need to clarify roles and practices in conjunction with other health professions to ensure the delivery of optimum health care and the need for increased financial support for nurses and nursing so that appropriate numbers and kinds of nurses are prepared to meet present and future demands for quality health care in the years to come.[3]

Considering the resolutions and recommendations that point to the future focus for nurses and nursing, it appears that nurses will be intellectually, interpersonally, and technically busy. The nursing process, as the key to quality nursing practice, will be an important part of future nursing practice.

To conclude our presentation on the nursing process, we would like to repeat this often-quoted story: A chicken and a pig were walking down the street. As they walked they came to a billboard displaying a breakfast of ham and eggs. The chicken said to the pig: "Look at the wonderful contribution I have made to mankind." The pig listened, then said: "Yes, that's fine, but my contribution involves a total commitment!"

REFERENCES

1. The stormy 70's—big changes still to come. Changing Times 26:25-31, 1972
2. Toffler A: Future Shock, part 1. New York, Random House, 1970, pp 1-50
3. Lysaught J: An Abstract for Action. New York, McGraw-Hill, 1970, pp 84-155
4. Fox D: Fundamentals of Research in Nursing. Second edition. New York, Appleton-Century-Crofts, 1970, pp 52-67
5. Ardrey R: The Territorial Imperative. New York, Atheneum, 1966, pp 1-155
6. Sommer, R, Dewar R: The physical environment of the ward, The Hospital in Modern Society. Edited by E. Freidson. New York, Free Press of Glencoe, 1963
7. Crenshaw A E: Invasion of Personal Space as Perceived by a Selected Group of Patients. Unpublished Masters Dissertation, School of Nursing, The Catholic University of America, Washington DC, May 1972
8. ANA convention. Am J Nurs 72:1102-114, 1972
9. NLN-NSNA convention, 1971. Nurs Outlook 14:390-409, 1971

APPENDIX A

THE CODE FOR NURSES*

1. The nurse provides services with respect for the dignity of man, unrestricted by considerations of nationality, race, creed, color, or status.
2. The nurse safeguards the individual's right to privacy by judiciously protecting information of a confidential nature, sharing only that information relevant to his care.
3. The nurse maintains individual competence in nursing practice, recognizing and accepting responsibility for individual actions and judgments.
4. The nurse acts to safeguard the patient when his care and safety are affected by incompetent, unethical, or illegal conduct of any person.
5. The nurse uses individual competence as a criterion in accepting delegated responsibilities and assigning nursing activities to others.
6. The nurse participates in research activities when assured that the rights of individual subjects are protected.
7. The nurse participates in the efforts of the profession to define and upgrade standards of nursing practice and education.
8. The nurse, acting through the professional organization, participates in establishing and maintaining conditions of employment conducive to high-quality nursing care.
9. The nurse works with members of health professions and other citizens in promoting efforts to meet the health needs of the public.
10. The nurse refuses to give or imply endorsement to advertising, promotion, or sales for commercial products, services, or enterprises.

*American Nurses' Association. Code for Nurses. Am J Nurs 68:2581-2585, 1968

APPENDIX B

List of observations that can be made by the nurse through the use of her four senses—seeing, hearing, smelling, and touching.

I. Observations Made by Seeing
  a. The Client
    1. General appearance and visible mood expression. Male, female, infant, child, adolescent, young adult, middle-aged adult, older adult, aged, estimation of age, age appropriateness, younger-appearing, older-appearing, tall, slim, short, malnourished, obese, plump, wasting, lean, thin, sad, happy, bored, anxious, fearful, eager, alert, attentive, sleepy, staring, tearful, frowning, inattentive, nervous, depressed, hyperactive, conscious, preoccupied, comatose, unconscious, nonresponsive.
    2. Visible physical factors
      a. Head and neck area: macrocephalic, microcephalic, normocephalic, goiter, tumors, swelling, infections, tics, paralysis, stiffness, congenital malformations, scars, hematoma
      b. Hair: amount, distribution, color—natural, dyed; baldness—scattered, circumscribed, extensive; long, short, straight, braided, curled, coiffeured, bearded, mustache, simply combed, unkempt, oily, lice, ringworm, hair cosmetics and jewelry, hairpieces, wigs, dandruff
      c. Eyes: strabismus, tearing, swollen lids, ecchymotic, clear, reddened, eye makeup, shaggy eyebrows, tweezed eyebrows; ptosis of lids—symmetric, unequal; bulging eyes, slanted eyes, squinting eyes, puffy lids, photophobic eyes, cataracts, blinking, eyeglasses, contact lenses, artificial eyes; pupils—regular, irregular, dilated, contracted; blind, twitching, sleeping
      d. Nose: small, pugnosed, enlarged, distorted, draining—mucus, blood, purulent; normal septum, septal deviation; tumors, dilated nares, pinched nares
      e. Ears: normal, enlarged, small, absent, deformed—congenital, cauliflower; drainage—bloody, purulent,

waxy; swelling in front of and/or behind, pierced ears, earrings

f. Lips, mouth, and teeth: protruding tongue, protruding teeth, full dentition—primary, secondary; lips—moist, parched, cracked; coated tongue, presence of food, gum, tobacco, toys in mouth; dentures—partial, full; missing unreplaced teeth, stained teeth—tea, coffee, tobacco, drugs: fillings—minimal, copious, crowns, caps, gold; hairlip, cleft palate—repaired, unrepaired, twitching, scars, distorted configuration, chancre, vomiting—projectile; air swallowing, mouth breathing, normal breathing, difficult breathing, drooling, herpes simplex, tumors, swelling, paralysis, lipstick, eating, drinking, yawning, sneezing, sordes, teeth chattering

g. Skin: clear, blushing, bruised, cuts, scratches, abrasions, fistulae, sinuses; elevations—tumors, warts, blisters, boils, carbuncles, abscesses, pimples, pustules, hives, pox, papules; chafed, sunburn, burns, flaking, peeling, rashes—circumscribed, profuse, generalized; acne, hemorrhage, scars, punctures, vaccination scar, venipuncture, venipuncture scars; color—racial, nationality, hereditary; pathologic color—jaundice, pallor, waxy, cyanotic, mottling; goose flesh; infestation—pin worms, lice; drainage—serous, serosanguinous, bloody, mucus, purulent; callouses, corns, bunions, tattoos, attached umbilical cord, healed umbilicus, dehydrated; soiled—urine, blood, feces, purulent material, dirt, other substances as tar, adhesive marks; discolored—gentian violet, potassium permanganate, silver nitrate, tincture of benzoin; presence of powders, pastes, deodorants, keloid, tumor, hernia, decubiti, ulcers, radiation markings, sutures, diaper rash, prickly heat

h. Posture: position; erect, upright, straight without support, straight with support—braces, cane, crutches, walker; distorted—kyphosis, lordosis, scoliosis, wrenched; pacing, rigid, shuffling gait, foot dragging; sitting—legs and feet relaxed, knees crossed, ankles crossed, swinging legs, in chair, on floor, in wheelchair, on edge of bed; dorsal recumbent, side lying, supine, prone, jackknife, opisthotonos, Fowler's, semi-Fowler's, dorsal lithotomy, knee-chest, immobile, mobile; walking—slowing, rapidly, limping; shivering, kneeling, squatting, jumping, creeping, crawling, running, fainting, sleep walking, convulsing, writhing, unusual position, palsied, shaking chills, stiffness

i. Extremities: extended, paralyzed, absence of portion (fingers, toes) or all of extremity, contractures, foot drop, hand drop, artificial limb, mongoloid palm, asymmetry, extra gluteal fold, wringing hands, tapping feet, kicking, crippled, clubfoot, knockknees, hairy; stained extremities—occupational dyes, tar, nicotine; fingernails, toenails—short, manicured, long, dirty, bitten, hangnails, blood blister, cracked, chipped, absent; arch supports, corrective shoes, bunions, barefeet, unequal limb length, bow legs, excessive muscle development, minimal muscle development, dislocation, fractures—green stick, compound; gangrene, parts cut out of shoes, bandages, bandaids, clenched fist, clutching items, clean hands and feet, soiled hands—dirt, blood, body secretions; tremors, twitching, flapping, picking, pushing, holding, clapping, patting, scratching, touching, frostbitten, left-handed, right-handed, ambidextrous

j. Trunk area: rhythmic breathing, barrel chest, protruding ribs, absence of rib, scars, tumors, burns, abrasions, lacerations, swelling, distortions, discolorations; breasts—developing, mature, male, female, enlarged, symmetric, asymmetric, lactating; nipples—normal nonparous, parous, cracked, inverted, bleeding, absence of breast; colostomy, gastrostomy, ileostomy; abdomen—flat, protruding, distended, obese, pregnant; scars, striae; back—spina bifida, pilonidal sinus; hemorrhage, incisions, puncture; hernia—umbilical, inguinal, incisional

k. Pelvic and genital area: male, female, infant, child, adolescent, adult, congenital anomalies; discharges—normal, pathogenic; tumors, swelling, menstruating, diaper, incontinent, infant stool—meconium, yellow, green; bloody urine, constipated stool, diarrhea, tumor, abscesses, lacerations, abrasions, urine and stool abnormalities—blood (red and tarry), worms, stones, undigested food; vaginal hemorrhage, bloody show, amniotic fluid

3. Clothing. Work clothes, fully clad, underclothing, naked, mod clothing, summer light clothing, heavy winter clothing—appropriate and inappropriate to climate; heavy socks, multiple pairs of socks, gloves, business dress, uniform, nightwear—pajamas, nightgown; formal evening wear, clean, soiled, wet, buttons and zippers closed, buttons and zippers opened, diaper, bunting, cultural and national variation, religious garb, bedroom slippers, rubbers, boots, masculine clothing, feminine clothing, institutional clothing, personal clothing

4. Attachments and prostheses. Jewelry, wedding band, rings, watches, eyeglasses—bifocals, trifocals, sunglasses, tinted glasses; contact lenses, hearing aids, dentures, bridgework, bandages, dressings, slings, colostomy bag, ileostomy bag, artificial limbs, facial prostheses, catheters—chest, bladder, drains, intubation—gastric, chest, tracheostomy, gastrostomy, intestinal, rectal; dressings—heavy, absorbent, sponges, bandaid, adhesive butterfly, improvised bandage, ace bandage; support hose, support socks, heel and elbow protectors, restraints, infusions—venous, peritoneal, dialysis; monitor leads, EEG and EKG lead attachments, blood pressure cuff; crutches, canes, walkers, wheelchair, corrective shoes, urinary bag—internal, external; vaginal pads, tampons, trusses, braces—teeth, extremities, pelvic, back; sutures, casts, compresses, heating pads, hot water bottle

b. External Environment of the Client

1. Immediate: personal possession—wallet, purse, blanket, pictures, luggage, books, newspaper, letters, brief case, toilet articles, easy chair, denture cup, toys; room—small, large, medium; room location—health care facility, home, school, campus, industry, migrant camp, nursery, clinic, single home, townhouse, high rise apartment, home for the aged, mobile home, shack; type of room—

bathroom, kitchen, living room, garage; furnishings—type, number, absence of; presence of other persons—parents, husband, wife, children, neighbors, friends, clergy, lawyer, police, other relatives, strangers, co-workers, colleagues, health care personnel, total number of persons

2. Neighborhood: urban, rural, inner city, suburbs, industrial, retirement community, college town, military installation, homeowners, rentals, young adults, river or harbor town, resort, paved, unpaved, lawns, tree-lined streets, absence of shrubbery, successful stores, well-designed store fronts, deteriorated business area, many vacancies, boarded-up store fronts, flowers, shrubs, trees, lawns, dusty, litter, parks, playground; available services within one block or within walking distances—grocery store, supermarket, speciality stores, delicatessen, bakery, laundry and cleaners, bookstore, shoe repair, physician and dentist offices, schools, church, police department, fire department, ambulance service; health care facilities—outpatient and inpatient, public transportation; heavy traffic, light traffic, museums, theaters, liquor stores, cocktail lounges, bars, coffee houses, pool halls, athletic associations, bowling alleys, street lighting, emergency call system, suicide prevention center, lighted hallways, elevators, indoor plumbing, bathroom—individual, shared; refrigerator, disposal of waste—disposals, garbage cans; pets—dogs, cats, other; presence or absence of flies, rodents, mosquitos, heat, air conditioning, handrailings on stairways, rugs, wooden floors, dirt floors

II. Observations Made by Hearing
  a. The Client
  1. Voice and speech: calm, excited, demanding, verbal messages—expressions of need, problems, hopes, fears, concerns, attitude, pain, verbal expressions of identification and orientation, requests for items, services, people, companionship, love, care; soft, inaudible, loud, jargon, crying, laughing, face-to-face conversation, telephone conversation, masculine, feminine, stammering, eructation, hiccough, burping, esophageal speech, unintelligible speech, strained, whispering, hoarse, stuttering, tongue-

tied, slurred, lisp, foreign language, snoring, aphasic, singing, grunting, silent, dialect—local, regional, national; vernacular, moaning, muffled, babbling, screeching, gasping

2. Breathing: rhythmic, slow, rapid, shallow, deep, stertorous, Cheyne-Stokes, apnea, wheezing, whistling, blowing, diverted through tracheostomy, coughing, sneezing, hiccoughing, gasping, burping, panting, rales, noisy

3. Heart sounds: apex rate—regular beat, irregular beat, tachycardia, bradycardia; murmur, absence of sound

4. Abdomen: presence of peristalsis, hyperactive peristalsis, hypoactive peristalsis, absence of peristalsis, flatus

b. Environment

1. Immediate: dripping, clicking, sucking, conversation with client and/or in the vicinity of client, traffic, public address system, laughing, absence of sound; radio, television, phonograph sounds, noises—squeaks, banging, clanging, knocking, dishes, carts, utensils, elevators, stairs

2. Neighborhood: traffic—heavy, light, distressful—ambulance sirens, police sirens, fire engines; trains, airplanes, car horns, animals—dogs, cats, farm animals, birds and wild animals; music—soft, rock and roll, mixed, loud, popular, life, recorded; children's voices, crying, screaming, calling, telephones, knocking, radio and television, phonograph, church bells, industrial sounds, bumping, hammering, sawing, pulling and pushing items and carts

III. Observations Made by Touching

a. The Client—body contour, size

1. Hair: dry, coarse, soft, fine, baby fine

2. Skin: smooth, clammy, rough, moist, dry, lumps, tumors, warts, moles, abscesses, edema, cold, cool, warm, hot; pulsations—regular, irregular, intermittent, strong, weak, scarcely perceptible, thready; goose flesh, painful, swelling

·3. Chest: expansion and relaxation, masses, painful areas, breast—lumps, engorged, size; brachial, carotid, radial, temporal, femoral, pedal, popliteal, facial pulses, enlarged axillary nodes

4. Abdomen: soft, hard, masses, tumors, distended, flat full urinary bladder, gaseous abdomen, painful,

herniation, taut, uterine contractions

5. Dressings: wet, dry
6. Bedding: wet, dry, damp, saturated, warm, cold
7. Muscle tension: muscle relaxation, throbbing, chills, twitching, spasm, convulsing, tremors, tumors, tics, firmness and fit of prostheses

b. Environment

Temperature and humidity of immediate environment, outdoor temperature and humidity; presence or absence of supports and railings, fences, bedsides

IV. Observations Made by Smelling

a. The Client

Perspiration, body odor, foot odor, axillary odor, pubic odor, hair odor—oily, perfumes, hairdressing; breath odor—sweet, alcohol, musty, tobacco, onion, garlic, commercial gargles, fetid, spicy, aromatic, pungent; bodily discharges—feces, urine, vomitus, purulent, necrotic, burned skin, burned or singed hair; use of chemicals—iodoform, liniments, ointments, anesthetics, antiseptics

b. Environment

Food odors: vegetables, fruits, meat, charcoal pit, barbecue, condiments, spices, coffee, restaurant odor, bakery, decaying food; exhaust—traffic, industrial odors, hospital odors, burning leaves, gas odors; odor of deodorants—pine oil, lysol, soap, peppermint; laboratory odors—antiseptics, cleaning materials, sprays; flowers, shrubs, hay, mowed lawn, farm odors, animal odors—skunk, dog, cat, horse

BIBLIOGRAPHY

GENERAL REFERENCES

BOOKS

Abdellah F, Beland I, Martin A, et al: Patient-Centered Approaches to Nursing. New York, The Macmillan Company, 1960

Aguilera D, Messick J, Farrell M: Crisis-Intervention, Theory and Methodology. St. Louis, CV Mosby, 1970

Anderson B: The Psychology Experiment. Second edition. Belmont, Calif, Brooks/Cole Publishing Company, 1971

Ardrey R: The Territorial Imperative. New York, Atheneum, 1966

A Sociological Framework for Patient Care. Edited by J Folta, E Deck. New York, John Wiley and Sons, Inc, 1966

Barnard C: The Functions of the Executive. Cambridge, Harvard University Press, 1964

Bermosk I S, Mordan M J: Interviewing in Nursing. New York, The Macmillan Company, 1964

Brown E L: Nursing For the Future. New York, Russell Sage Foundation, 1948

Idem: Newer Dimensions of Patient Care, parts 1, 2, and 3. New York, Russel Sage Foundation, 1964

Brown M, Fowler G: Psychodynamic Nursing. Fourth edition. Philadelphia, WB Saunders Co, 1971

Buber, M: The Knowledge of Man. New York, Harper and Row, 1965

Idem: I and Thou. Second edition. New York, Charles Scribner's Sons, 1958

Continuity of Patient Care: The Role of Nursing. Proceedings of the Workshop. Edited by K M Straub, K S Parker. Washington, DC, The Catholic University of America Press, 1966

Copi I: Introduction to Logic. Second edition. New York, The Macmillan Company, 1961

Dubos R: Man Adapting. New Haven, Yale University Press, 1965

Dunn H L: High-Level Wellness. Arlington, Va, Beatty Company, 1967

Fast J: Body Language. New York, M Evans and Co, 1970

Frank C M: Foundations of Nursing. Philadelphia, WB Saunders Co, 1959, p78

Frankl V: Man's Search for Meaning. New York, Washington Square Press, 1963

Hadley B J: Evolution of a conception of nursing. Nurs Res 18:400-404, 1969

Jaco E: Patients, Physicians and Illness. Glencoe, Ill, Free Press, 1958

Jourard S M: The Transparent Self. Princeton, New Jesrey, Van Nostrand, 1964

Kuethe J: The Teaching-Learning Process. Glenview, Ill, Scott, Freemand and Company, 1968

Lachman S: The Foundation of Science. New York, Vantage Press, Inc, 1960

Leavell H, Clark E G: Preventive Medicine for the Doctor in His Community. Third edition. New York, McGraw-Hill Publishing Company, 1966

Lysaught J: Abstract for Action. New York, McGraw-Hill Publishing Co, 1970

Mager R: Goal Analysis. Belmont, Calif, Fearon Publishers, 1972

Maslow A H: Motivation and Personality. New York, Harper and Brothers, 1954

Idem: Toward A Psychology of Being. Second edition. Princeton, New Jersey, Van Nostrand, 1968

McCaffery M: Nursing Management of the Patient with Pain. Philadelphia, JB Lippincott Co, 1972

Meyer B, Heidgerken L E: Introduction to Research in Nursing. Philadelphia, JB Lippincott Co, 1962

Nightingale F: Notes on Nursing: What It Is and What It Is Not. A facsimile of the first edition published in 1859. Philadelphia, JB Lippincott Co, 1946

Nordmark M, Rohweder A: Science Foundations of Nursing. Philadelphia, JB Lippincott Co, 1967

Peter L J, Hull R: The Peter Principle. New York, William Morrow and Co, Inc, 1969

Pohl M: Teaching Function of the Nursing Practitioner. Dubuque, Iowa, Wm C Brown Co, 1968

Simon H: The Sciences of the Artificial. Cambridge, The MIT Press, 1969

Smith D W: Medical-Surgical Nursing in the Curriculum—Purpose and Process, Curriculum and Instruction in Medical - Surgical and Psychiatric Nursing in Baccalaureate Programs. Edited by V Conley. Washington, DC, Catholic University of America Press, 1970

Social Interaction and Patient Care. Edited by JK Skipper, RC Leonard. Philadelphia, JB Lippincott Co, 1965

The Nursing Profession: Five Sociological Essays. Edited by F Davis. New York, John Wiley and Sons, Inc, 1966

Toffler A: Future Shock. New York, Random House, Inc, 1970

Toward Quality in Nursing, Needs and Goals. Washington, DC, Public Health Service, US Department of Health, Education, and Welfare, 1963

Travelbee J: Interpersonal Aspects of Nursing. Second edition. Philadelphia, FA Davis Co, 1971

Ujhely G B: Determinants of the Nurse-Patient Relationship. New York, Springer Publishing Co, 1968

Walker V: Nursing and Ritualistic Practice. New York, The Macmillan Co, 1967

Wensley E: Nursing Service Without Walls—A Call to Action to All Communities Coast to Coast. New York, National League for Nursing, Inc, 1963

COMMUNICATION

Ackoff R: Towards a behavioral theory of communication, In Modern Systems Research for the Behavioral Scientist. Edited by W Buckley. Chicago, Aldine Press, 1968, pp 209-218

Bonkovsky M: Adapting the POMR to community child health care. Nurs Outlook 20:515-518, 1972

Calnan M F, Hanrow J B: Patient-centered communication. Supervisor Nurse 2:67-71, 1971

Ellis L: Communications and interdepartmental relationships. Nurs Forum 5:82-89, 1966

Healy E, McGurk W: Effectiveness and acceptance of nurses' notes. Nurs Outlook, 14:32-34, 1966

Hewitt H E, Pesznecker B L: Blocks of communicating with patients. Am Nurs 64:101-103, 1964

The Problem-Oriented System. Edited by J Hurst and HK Walker. New York, Medcom Press, 1972

Kron T: Communication in nursing. Philadelphia, WB Saunders Co, 1972

Lewis G: Communication: a factor in meeting emotional crises. Nurs Outlook 13:36-39, 1965

Idem: Nurse-Patient Communication. Dubuque, Iowa, Wm C Brown Co, 1969

Raymond R: Communication, entropy, and life, Modern Systems Research for the Behavioral Scientist. Buckley W (ed),[1] pp 157-160

Schell P, Campbell A: POMR—Not just another way to chart. Nurs Outlook 20:510-514

Theis C, Harrington H: Three factors that affect practice—communications, assignments, attitudes. Am J Nurs 68:1478-1482, 1968

Weed L: Medical Records, Medical Education, and Patient Care. Cleveland, Press of Case Western Reserve University, 1970

FILM

The Pulses Profile. New York State Department of Health, 1970, 16 mm; American Journal of Nursing Film Library, c/o Association-Sterling Films, 600 Grand Avenue, Ridgefield, New Jersey, 07657

GENERAL THEORY

Administrative Theory in Education. Edited by A Halpin. London, Macmillan Co, 1958

Allport G: The open system in personality theory, Modern Systems Research for the Behavioral Scientist. Edited by Walter Buckley. Chicago, Aldine Publishing Co, 1968, pp 343-350

Banathy B H: Instructional Systems. Fearon Publishers, Palo Alto, California, 1968

Bertalanffy L von: General System Theory. New York, George Braziller, Inc, 1968

Idem: General system theory—a critical review.[2] pp 11-30

Boulding K: General system theory—the skeleton of science.[2] pp 3-10

Frick F C: The application of information theory in behavioral studies.[2] pp 182-185

Griffiths D: Administrative Theory. New York, Appleton-Century-Crofts, Inc, 1959

Hall A D, Fagen R E: Definition of system.[2] pp 81-92

Hazzard M: An overview of systems theory. Nurs Clin N Am 6:385-393, 1971

Mackay D: The informational analysis of questions and commands.[2] pp 204-208

Idem: Towards an information-flow model of human behavior.[2] pp 395-368

Miller G A: What is information measurement?[2] pp 123-128

Modern Systems Research for the Behavioral Scientist. Edited by W Buckley. Chicago, Aldine Publishing Co, 1968

Rapoport A, Horvath W: Thoughts on organizational theory.[2] pp 71-75

Idem: Critiques of game theory.[2] pp 474-489

Idem: The promise and pitfalls of information theory.[2] pp 137-142

Raymond R: Communication, entropy, and life.[2] pp 157-165

Schimpf K: The human body as an energy system. Am J Nurs 71:117-120, 1971

Schrödinger E: Order, disorder, and entropy.[2] pp 143-146

Slack C: Feedback theory and the reflex arc concept.[2] pp 317-320

Society as a complex adaptive system.[2] pp 490-513

Symposium on a systems approach to nursing. Nurs Clin N Am 6:383-462, 1971

Tomotsu S: A cybernetic approach to motivation.[2] pp 330-336

[2] Chapter in Buckley W ed: Modern Systems Research for the Behavioral Scientist. Chicago, Aldine Publishing Co, 1968

LEADERSHIP

Dietrich J, Miller I: Nursing leadership—a theoretical framework. Nurs Outlook 14:52-55, 1966

Douglass L, Bevis Em O: Team leadership in action. St Louis, CV Mosby Co, 1970

Mercadante L T: Leadership development seminars. Nurs Outlook, 13:59-61, 1965

Merton R: The social nature of leadership. Am J Nurs 69:2614-2618, 1969

The Assessment of Leader Behaviors. Sigma Theta Tau, First Regional Conference, Storrs, Connecticut, Sigma Theta Tau, 1969

Yura H: Nursing leadership behavior. Supervisor Nurs 2:55-64, 1971

NURSING ASSESSMENT

Black M K: Assessing patient's needs, The Nursing Process. Edited by H Yura, M Walsh. Washington, DC, The Catholic University of America Press, 1967, pp 1-20

Dahlin B: Rehabilitation and the assessment of patient need. Nurs Clin N Am 1:375-386, 1966

Family Coping Index, Developed by Johns Hopkins School of Hygiene and Public Health and Richmond Instructive Visiting Nurse Association—City Health Department, Nursing Service (Richmond-Hopkins Cooperative Nursing Study), Directed by R B Freeman, 1964

Gilbo D: Nursing assessment of circulatory function. Nurs Clin N Am 3:53-64, 1968

Haferkorn V: Assessing individual learning needs as a basis for patient teaching. Nurs Clin N Am 6:199-209, 1971

Hamilton C, Pratt M, Groen M: The nurses' active role in assessment. Nurs Clin N Am 4:249-262, 1969

Harpine F: Assessing the Needs of the Patient, The Nursing Process. Yura H, Walsh M, (eds.),[1] pp 21-49

Huang S H: Nursing assessment in planning care for a diabetic patient. Nurs Clin N Am 6:135-143, 1971

Jackson E B: In the screening clinics, guidelines to the appraisal of some common problems. Am J Nurs 72:1398-1400, 1972

Levine M: Adaptation and assessment: a rationale for nursing intervention. Am J Nurs 66:2450-2453, 1966

McCain F: Nursing by assessment, not intuition. Am J Nurs 65:82-84, 1965

Peabody S: Assessment and planning for continuity of care from hospital to home. Nurs Clin N Am:303-310, 1969

Peterson L W: Operant approach to observation and recording. Nurs Outlook 15:28-32, 1967

Poland M: A system for assessing and meeting patient needs. Am J Nurs 70:1479-1482, 1970

NURSING AUDIT

Carn I: The nursing audit as a learning tool for undergraduates in the community nursing services. Nurs Clin N Am 4:351-358, 1969

McGuire R L: Bedside nursing audit. Am J Nurs 68:2146-2148, 1968

Planeuf M: A nursing audit method. Nurs Outlook 12:42-45, 1964

Idem: The nursing audit for evaluation of patient care. Nurs Outlook 14:51-54, 1966

Idem: The Nursing Audit. New York, Appleton-Century-Crofts, 1972

NURSING CARE PLANS

Cornell S, Brush F: Systems approach to nursing care plans. Am J Nurs 71:1376-1378, 1971

Drucker P F: The effective decision. Harvard Business Review Jan-Feb 1967, pp 92-98

Harmer B: Methods and Principles of Teaching the Principles and Practice of Nursing. New York, Macmillan Co, 1926

Hickox L: Planning to Meet Patient Needs. The Nursing Process. Edited by H Yura, M Walsh. Washington, DC, The Catholic University of America Press, 1967, pp 60-77

Kelly N: Nursing care plans. Nurs Outlook 14:61-64, 1966

Lambertsen E: Nursing care plan should reflect present and future patient needs. Mod Hosp 103:128, 1964

Lewis L: Planning Patient Care. Dubuque, Iowa, Wm C Brown Co, 1970

Little D, Carnevali D: Nursing Care Planning. Philadelphia, JB Lippincott Co, 1969

Mansfield E: Care plans to stimulate learning. Am J Nurs 68:2592-2593, 1968

Mayers M: A Systematic Approach to the Nursing Care Plan. New York, Appleton-Century-Crofts, 1972

Nettleton J: Planning to meet patient needs. The Nursing Process,[4] pp 44-59

Patterson E A, Stence F L: Thinking together to solve care problems. Am J Nurs 70:1703-1706, 1970

Smith D M: Writing objectives as a nursing practice skill. Am J Nurs 71:319-320, 1971

Wagner B: Care plans—right, reasonable, and reachable. Am J Nurs 69:986-990, 1969

Walker V, Mc Reynolds D, Patrick E: A care plan for ailing nurses' notes. Am J Nurs 65:74-76, 1965

NURSING DEFINITION

Coladarci A P: What about that word profession? Am J Nurs 63:116-118, 1963

Flexner A: Universities. New York, Oxford University Press, 1930, pp 29-30

Hall L E: Quality of Nursing Care. Address at meeting of Department of Baccalaureate and Higher Degree Programs of the New Jersey League for Nursing, February 7, 1955, Seton Hall University, Newark, New Jersey. Published in Public Health News, New Jersey State Department of Health, June, 1955

Idem: A center for nursing. Nurs Outlook 11:805-806, 1963

Henderson V: The nature of nursing. Am J Nurs 64:62-68, 1964

Idem: The Nature of Nursing. New York, The Macmillan Co, 1966

Idem: Excellence in nursing. Am J Nurs 69:2133-2137, 1969

Johnson M M, Martin H W: A sociological analysis of the nurse role. Am J Nurs 58:373-377, 1958

Johnson D E: Today's action will determine tomorrow's nursing. Nurs Outlook 13:38-41, 1965

Idem: The significance of nursing care. Am J Nurs 61:63-66, 1961

Kreuter F R: What is good nursing care? Nurs Outlook 5:302-304, 1957

Lambertsen E C: Nursing definition and philosophy precede nursing goal development. Mod Hosp 103:136, 1964

Orem D: The hope of nursing. J Nurs Educ 1:5-7, 1962

Idem: Nursing: Concepts of Practice. New York, McGraw-Hill Book Co, 1971

Poland M, English N, Thornton N, Owens D: PETO—A system for assessing and meeting patient care needs. Am J Nurs 70:1479-1482, 1970

Reiter F: Nurse clinician. Am J Nurs 66:274-278, 1966
Idem: Choosing the better part. Am J Nurs 64:65-68
Rushing W: The hospital nurse as a mother surrogate and bedside psychologist. Ment Hyg 50:71-79, 1966
Schmidt J: Availability: a concept of nursing practice. Am J Nurs 72:1086-1089, 1972
Wiedenbach E: Clinical Nursing: A Helping Art. New York, Springer Publishing Co, 1964
Idem: The helping art of nursing. Am J Nurs 63:54-57, 1963
Whiting F J: Patient's needs, nurse's needs and the healing process. Am J Nurs 58:661-665, 1958

NURSING DIAGNOSIS

Bonney V, Rothberg J: Nursing Diagnosis and Therapy—An Instrument for Evaluation and Measurement. New York, The League Exchange, National League for Nursing, 1963
Chambers W: Nursing diagnosis. Am J Nurs 62:102-104, 1962
Durand M, Prince R: Nursing Diagnosis: process and decision. Nurs Forum 5:50-64, 1966
Hornung G J:The nursing diagnosis—an exercise in judgment? Nurs Outlook 4:29-30, 1956
Komorita N I: Nursing diagnosis. Am J Nurs 63:83-86, 1963
Rothberg J S: Why nursing diagnosis? Am J Nurs 67:1040-1042, 1967

NURSING EVALUATION

Abdellah F G, Levine E: Polling patients and personnel—Part I: What patients say about their nursing care. Hospitals 31:44-48, 1957
Abdellah F G: Criterion measures in nursing. Nurs Res 10:21-26, 1961
Agnus M: Evaluation: a constructive or a destructive force? Can Nurs 62:26-28, 1966
Butler J, Flood F R: Evaluating nursing care in a mental hospital. Am J Nurs 62:84-85, 1962
Clissold G, Metz E: Evaluation—a tangible process. Nurs Outlook 14:41-45, 1966
Cochran C, Hansen P J: Developing an evaluation tool by group action. Am J Nurs 62:94-96, 1962
Fivars G, Gosnell D: Nursing Evaluation: The Problem and the Process. New York, Macmillan Company, 1966
Lambertsen E: Evaluating the quality of nursing care. Hospitals 39:61-66, 1965
National League for Nursing. Evaluation—The Whys and The Ways. New York, The National League for Nursing, 1965
National League for Nursing. Quest for Quality: A Self Evaluation Guide to Patient Care. Prepared by Committee on Quality of Patient Care, Department of Hospital Nursing. New York, National League for Nursing, 1966

O'Shea H S: A guide to evaluation of clinical performance. Am J Nurs 67:1877-1879, 1967

Rosen A: Performance appraisal interviewing evaluated by professional observers. Nurs Res 16:32-37, 1967

Rosen A, Abraham G E: Evaluation of a procedure for assessing the performance of staff nurses. Nurs Res 12:78-82, 1963

St. Denis H: Evaluating the plan of care, The Nursing Process. Yura H, Walsh M (eds) Wash DC, Cath U Am Press 1967 pp 95-109

Swartz D: Toward more precise evaluation of patient's needs. Nurs Outlook 13:42-44, 1965

Woods M F: Measuring a patient's needs and progress. Nurs Outlook 14:38-41, 1966

Wood V: Measurement and evaluation in nursing education. Can Nurse 62:54-58, 1966

NURSING HISTORY

Gangwer M E: Identification of Crucial Information for a Nursing History. Unpublished Masters Dissertation, Washington, DC, The Catholic University of America, School of Nursing, 1965

McPhettridge L M: Nursing history: one means to personalize care. Am J Nurs 68:68-75

Smith D: A clinical nursing tool. Am J Nurs 68:2384-2388

NURSING PROCESS

American Nurses' Association. Standards for organized nursing services. Am J Nurs 65:76-79

Bailey D E: Clinical inference in nursing: Analysis of Nursing Action Patterns. Nurs Res 16:154-160, 1967

Baldridge P: The nurse in triage. Nurs Outlook 14:46-48, 1966

Barckley V: Enough time for good nursing. Nurs Outlook 12:44-48, 1964

Barrett-Lennard G T: Significant aspects of a helping relationship. Canada's Ment Health Special Suppl 47: 1-5, 1965

Burrill M: Helping students identify and solve patients' problems. Nurs Outlook 14:46-48, 1966

Byers V: Nursing Observation. Dubuque, Iowa, Wm C Brown Co, 1968

Campbell M: Identifying nursing problems. Can Nurse 61:96-99, 1965

Carrieri V K, Sitzman J: Components of the nursing process. Nurs Clin N Am 6:115-124, 1971

Condon M B: Teaching the teachers. Nurs Outlook 19:804-806, 1971

Davitz L J, Pendleton S: Nurses' inferences of suffering. Nurs Res 18:100-107, 1969

Hammond K R, Kelly K, Schneider, R, et al: Clinical inference in nursing—analyzing cognitive tasks representative of nursing problems. Nurs Res 15:134-138, 1966

Hammond K R: Clinical inference in nursing—a psychologist's viewpoint. Nurs Res 15:27-38, 1966

Hammond K R, Kelly K J, Schneider R J, et al: Clinical inference in nursing—information units used. Nurs Res 15:236-243, 1966

Hammond K R, Kelly K, Castellan N J: Clinical inference in nursing: use of information seeking strategies by nurses. Nurs Res 15:330-336, 1966

Hammond K R, Kelly K, Schneider R: Clinical inference in nursing—revising judgments. Nurs Res 16:38-45, 1967

Harrison C: Deliberative nursing process versus automatic nurse action. Nurs Clin N Am 1:387-397, 1966

Hogan A I: The role of the nurse in meeting the needs of the new mother. Nurs Clin N Am 3:337-344, 1968

Hykawy E: A problem solving approach. Can Nurse 63:35-38, 1967

Jackson F B: In the screening clinic, guidelines to the appraisal of some common problems. Am J Nurs 72:1398-1400, 1972

Johnson M, Davis M I, Bilitch M: Problem-Solving in Nursing Practice. Dubuque, Iowa, Wm C Brown Co, 1970

Kelly K J, Hammond K: An approach to study of clinical inference in nursing. Nurs Res 13:314-322, 1964

Kelly K: Clinical inference in nursing—a nurse's viewpoint. Nurs Res 15:23-26, 1966

Kraegel J, Schmidt V, Shukla R, et al: A system of patient care based on patient needs. Nurs Outlook 20:257-264, 1972

Kramer M, Egan E, Knauber J: The effect of presets on creative problem solving. Nurs Res 19:303-311, 1970

Lewis L, Carozza V, Carroll M, et al: Defining Clinical Content Graduate Nursing Programs, Medical/Surgical Nursing. Boulder, Colorado: Western Interstate Commission for Higher Education, February, 1967

Lewis L: This I believe . . . about the nursing process—key to care. Nurs Outlook 16:26-29, 1968

McCaffery M, Moss F: Nursing intervention for bodily pain. Am J Nurs 67:1224-1227, 1967

Miller D I: Administration for the patient. Am J Nurs 65:114-116, 1965

Nadler G, Sahney V: A descriptive model of nursing care. Am J Nurs 69:336-341, 1969

Neshio K: Creative problem solving: a teaching innovation. Nurs Forum 6:432-441, 1967

Orlando I J: The Dynamic Nurse-Patient Relationship. New York, GP Putnam's Sons, 1961

Perrine G: Needs met and unmet. Am J Nurs 71:2128-2133, 1971

Price E: Data processing, present and potential. Am J Nurs 67:2558-2564, 1967

Standeven M: The relevant who of problem solving. Nurs Forum 10:166-175, 1971

Sutterly D, Donnelly G: Meeting nursing needs throughout the life cycle, chapter 3, Advanced Concepts in Clinical Nursing. Edited by K Kintzel. Philadelphia, JB Lippincott Co, 1971

Tapia J A: The nursing process in family health. Nurs Outlook 20:267-270, 1972

Taylor D B: A Clinical Information System: A Tool for Improving

Nurses' Decisions in Planning Patient Care. ANA Clinical Sessions, New York, Appleton-Century-Crofts, 1970, pp 159-169
The Nursing Process. Edited by H Yura, M Walsh. Washington, DC, The Catholic University of America Press, 1967
Wesolowski M: Implementing a plan of care. The Nursing Process. Edited by H Yura, M Walsh. Washington, DC, Catholic University of America Press, 1967
Zimmerman D S, Gohrke C: The goal-directed nursing approach: it does work. Am J Nurs 70:306-310, 1970

PERCEPTION

Allport F: Theories of Perception and the Concept of Structure. New York, John Wiley and Sons, 1955
Osgood C: A behavioristic analysis of perception and language as cognitive, Modern Systems Research for the Behavioral Scientist. Edited by W Buckley. Chicago, Aldine Publishing Co, 1968
Perceiving, Sensing, and Knowing. Edited by R Swartz. Garden City, New York, Anchor Books, Inc, 1965
Vernon M: Perception Through Experience. London, Methuen and Co, Ltd, 1970

PERIODICALS

Abdellah F: Criterion measures in nursing. Nurs Res 10:21-26, 1961
Alfano G: The Loeb Center for Nursing and Rehabilitation—a professional approach to nursing practice. Nurs Clin N Am 4:487-493, 1969
American Nurses' Association. Code for nurses. Am J Nurs 68:2581-2585, 1968
Bailey J T, McDonald F J, Calus K E: Evaluation of the development of creative behavior in an experimental nursing program. Nurs Res 19:100-108, 1970
Bates B, Kern M S: Doctor-nurse teamwork: what helps? What hinders? Am J Nurs 67:2066-2071, 1967
Brimigion J: Nursing administration in long-term care facilities: a dual-kardex system. J Nurs Administr 1:26-30, 1971
Brodt D: Obstacles to individualized patient care. Nurs Outlook 14:35-36, 1966
Donohue M A: The I-thou relationship. Nurs Outlook 14:59-61, 1966
Doxiadis C A: Man and the space around him. Saturday Review, December 14, 1968, pp 21-23
Dubos R: Man overadapting to the environment. Psychol Today 4:50-54, 1971
Establishing standards for nursing practice. Am J Nurs 69:1458-1463, 1969
Ellis R: The practitioner as theorist. Am J Nurs 69:1434-1438, 1969
Flanagan J: The critical incident technique. Psychol Bull 51:327-358, 1954

Greenough K: Determining standards for nursing care. Am J Nurs 68:2153-2157, 1968

Hall L: The Loeb Center for Nursing and Rehabilitation, Montefiore Hospital and Medical Center, Bronx, New York. Int J Nurs Studies 6:81-97, 1969

Idem: Another view of nursing care and quality. Maryland Nursing News (Spring), 1968, pp 2-12

MacGregor F: Uncooperative patients: some cultural interpretations. Am J Nurs 67:88-91, 1967

Minckley B B: Space and place in patient care. Am J Nurs 68:510-516, 1968

Murray R: Caring. Am J Nurs 72:1286-1287, 1972

Naugle E: Knock and wait. Am J Nurs 71:311-313, 1971

Newman M: Identifying and meeting patient's needs in short-span nurse-patient relationships. Nurs Forum 5:76-86, 1966

Palmer J: Management by objectives. J Nurs Administr 1:17-23, 1971

Parnes S J: Creativity: developing human potential. J Creative Behavior 5:19-36, 1971

Pluckhan M L: Space: The silent language. Nurs Forum 7:386-397, 1968

Quality patient care. Can Nurse 61:975-978, 1965

Ramphal M: The patient is the center of nursing. Maryland Nurs News (Spring) 1968, pp 13-20

The stormy 70's—big changes still to come. Changing Times. 26:25-31, 1972

Wolff I: Acceptance. Am J Nurs 72:1412-1415, 1972

PHILOSOPHY, SCIENCE OF NURSING, CONCEPTS, THEORIES OF NURSING

Abdellah F G: The nature of nursing science. Nurs Res 18:390-393, 1969

Arnold H M: I-Thou. Am J Nurs 70:2554-2556, 1970

Brodt D E: A synergistic theory of nursing. Am J Nurs 69:1674-1676, 1969

Brown M I: Research in the development of nursing theory. Nurs Res 13:109-112, 1964

Dickoff J, James P: A theory of theories: a position paper. Nurs Res 17:197-203, 1968

Ellis R: The practitioner as theorist. Am J Nurs 69:1434-1438, 1969

Halpert H P, Horvath W, Young J P: An Administrator's Handbook on the Application of Operations Research to the Management of Mental Health Systems. National Clearinghouse for Mental Health Information Public, No 1003, 1970

Hoffman G S: The concept of love. Nurs Clin N Am 4: 663-671, 1969

Horgan S M Visitation: Concepts About Nursing in Selected Nursing Literature from 1950-1965. Unpublished Masters Dissertation: Washington, DC, The Catholic University of America, School of Nursing, 1967

Johnson D: A philosophy of nursing. Nurs Outlook 7:198-200, 1969

Johnson D E: The nature of a science of nursing. Nurs Outlook 7:291-294, 1959

King I: a conceptual frame of reference for nursing. Nurs Res 17:27-31, 1968

Levine M E: The four conservation principles of nursing. Nurs Forum 6:45-59, 1967

McDonald F J, Harms M T: A theoretical model for an experimental curriculum. Nurs Outlook 14:48-51, 1966

McKay R P: The Process of Theory Development in Nursing. New York, Teachers College, Columbia University, A Report of an Ed D Doctoral Project, 1965

Miller D I: Administration for the patient. Am J Nurs 65:114-116, 1965

Murphy J F: Role expansion or role extension: some conceptual differences. Nurs Forum 9:380-390, 1970

Norris C: Toward a science of nursing. Nurs Forum 3:10-45, 1964

Newman M A: Nursing's theoretical evolution. Nurs Outlook 20:449-453, 1972

Reiter F: The nurse clinician. Am J Nurs 66:274-280

Theoretical Issues in Professional Nursing. Edited by J F Murphy. New York, Appleton-Century-Crofts Educational Division, Meredith Corp, 1971

Thigpen L A, Drane J W: The Venn diagram: a tool for conceptualization in nursing. Nurs Res 16:252-260, 1967

Vaillot M C: Existentialism: a philosophy of commitment. Am J Nurs 66:500-505, 1966

Idem: Nursing theory, levels of nursing, and curriculum development. Nurs Forum 9:234-249, 1970

Zderad L, Belcher H: Developing Behavioral Concepts in Nursing. Atlanta, Georgia, Southern Regional Education Board, 1968

Zderad L: Empathetic nursing. Nurs Clin N Am 4:655-662, 1969

SELECTED CLINICAL REFERENCES

Advanced Concepts in Clinical Nursing. Edited by K Kintzel. Philadelphia, JB Lippincott Co, 1971

Anonymous. Notes of a Dying Professor. Nurs Outlook 20:502-506, 1972

Crosby M: Control systems and children with lymphoblastic leukemia. Nurs Clin N Am 6:407-413, 1971

Francis G: Cancer: the emotional component. Am J Nurs 69:1677-1681, 1969

Griffiths E: Nursing process: a patient with a respiratory dysfunction. Nurs Clin N Am 6:145-154, 1971

Hodges L: Systems and nursing care of the cardiac surgical patient. Nurs Clin N Am 6:415-424, 1971

Jacobansky A: Strokes. Am J Nurs 72:1260-1263, 1972

Jaeger D, Simmons L: The Aged Ill. New York, Appleton-Century-Crofts, 1970

Kinney A B, Blount M: Systems approach to myasthenia gravis. Nurs Clin N Am 6:435-453, 1971

Levinger G, Billings H: Nursing in a low-rent housing project. Am J Nurs 71:315-318, 1971

Metheny N, Snively W D: Nurses' Handbook of Fluid Balance. Philadelphia, JB Lippincott Co, 1967

Miller J: Systems theory and family psychotherapy. Nurs Clin N Am 6:395-406, 1971

Moughton M: Systems and childhood psychosis. Nurs Clin N Am 6:425-434, 1971

Reres M: Systems analysis: an approach to working with personality disorders. Nurs Clin N Am 6:455-462, 1971

Shetler M: Operating room nurses go visiting. Am J Nurs 72:1266-1269, 1972

Slater M: Nursing intervention for the patient with central nervous system dysfunction, chap 16.[1] pp 368-409

Taylor D B: A clinical information system: a tool for improving nurses' decisions in planning patient care, ANA Clinical Sessions. New York, Appleton-Century-Crofts, 1970, pp 159-169

Warrick L: Family-centered care in the premature nursing. Am Nurs 71:2134,2138, 1971

Williams D: Sleep and disease. Am J Nurs 71:2321-2334, 1971

Worrell J: Nursing implication in the care of the patient experiencing sensory deprivation. Advanced Concepts in Clinical Nursing. Kintzel, K (ed).

Zborowski M: People in Pain. San Francisco, Jossey-Boss, Inc 1969

Index

Planning (*cont.*)
  definition of 28
  goals, types of 95–96
  horizontal 103
  orders, nursing 97–99
  and preplanning 105–7
  priorities, order of 93–95
  purpose of 93
  resources for 96
  situation report 102, 103
  vertical 103
  in wellness 93
Position paper, on education for
    nursing 8
Prejudices 61, 87
Preplanning 105–7
  in anticipated crises 106
  in case of fire 105
  for problem solving 105–6
Priority, setting of 93, 174
  agreement in 94
  client involvement in 94
  factors influencing 94
  high 93, 94
  low 94
  medium 94
  ordering of 95
Problem
  of client 104
  identification of 92
  judgments about 90–92
  legal 96
  spiritual 96
Problem-solving 47
Process, definition of 23
Profession
  criteria basic to 6
  nursing as a 6
Professional, use of term 5

Raymond, Richard 41
Recording 118
  automatic notations in 118
  frequency of 119
  indexing of 119
  profile of client in 119
  quality of 118

Research
  model for identification of
      problems for 177–78
  needs for, in nursing process
      136
  process 19, 177
  role
    in nursing process develop-
        ment 177
    in nursing science develop-
        ment 177
  studies 178–80

Self-development, of nurse 71
Sensory deprivation 55, 129
Sensory input 129
Simon, Herbert 47
Standards for nursing practice,
    development of 123
Suprasystem 37
System
  closed 64
  definition of 36
  living 40
  open 39, 40, 64

Technical skills 30, 69, 99, 120
Theory
  communication 35, 66
  cyclic nature of 65–66
  decision 35, 66
  general systems 35, 66
  information 35, 66
  of nursing 19
  of perception 35, 66
Toffler, Alvin 173
Touch 8, 195–96
Trust 24, 25

Vernon, Magdalen 55, 56, 57

Western Interstate Commission on
    Higher Education 21
Wiedenbach, Ernestine 12